The SEXY Diet
by Summer Peterson

Shrink Your Fat Cells,
Speed Up Your Metabolism
&
Activate Your Skinny Genes

Summer Peterson

ISBN: 9781719935050

The SEXY Diet

CONTENTS

ACKNOWLEDGMENTS

As an author, one learns early on that it takes a village to write a book. My village includes family, friends, clients, teachers and mentors. I am forever grateful for each and every one of these people who have inspired me, guided me and loved me through this process.

With each draft that I wrote, I felt my ancestor's guidance and felt them illuminate new ideas and uncover deep memories. These family members, whom I have not had the luxury of knowing in life, have had a strong impact on who I am and who I will become. Their voices can be felt in the stories I tell. Some of these ancestors were known to me and are now deceased, and I could feel their angelic love nurture me as I wrote.

I am profoundly grateful to the supportive team who made this book possible. Throughout this journey, each member of this team has become a genuine friend. I am deeply grateful to all of my friends who have believed in me every step of this process. I am blessed to have supportive friends that authentically celebrate my wins and I particularly enjoy celebrating their wins as well. Thank you for lifting me up and blessing me with the opportunity to lift you up too.

To the clients that have put their trust in me, I am forever grateful to you. I have learned invaluable lessons from witnessing your powerful transformations and I am deeply grateful to have received permission to write your stories in the pages of this book. It is your stories that will inspire the readers into their own profound transformations.

I have had countless teachers and mentors throughout my life, all of whom have made a significant impact on me, making this book possible. I crossed paths with many of these mentors years ago, but their influence is still powerfully felt. Some of these mentors do not even know I exist. They have all made me a better person and I would be remiss not to acknowledge them.

Lastly, from the depths of my heart and soul, I acknowledge my loving family. They are my greatest source of inspiration. They are my home. They are my deepest source of nourishment. To all of my family members, thank you for your kindness, your craziness and ever-present love. To my dear husband, I love you madly. To our amazing sons, Jude and Skyler, our hearts will forever beat in tune and my greatest joy is the love we share.

INTRODUCTION

Unleash the Sexy Beast Within

ALLOW ME TO INTRODUCE MYSELF

My name is Summer and I was born and raised in the heart of the Northern California Wine Country. My father grew grapes at some of the most prestigious, world renowned wineries in the Napa Valley, and my mother was an actress, writer and counselor.

I wasn't always overweight. I had been one of the lucky ones, relatively thin throughout my childhood and into my 20's. But my mother had always told me that once she hit 30, her metabolism had slowed down causing her to gain weight that she was never able to lose. Right around my 30th birthday, my mother's words became my reality. The weight seemed to come out of nowhere and I was miserable. I found myself 30 pounds heavier than I had ever been and I felt unlovable. Every time I looked in the mirror I felt shame and self-hatred.

I believed that I had inherited a metabolism that was programmed to slow down when I turned 30. I began to hate my body because I believed it was betraying me. I resented my family for giving me a genetic inheritance of an overweight body and a slow metabolism.

I WAGED WAR WITH MY METABOLISM

I desperately tried to lose the weight, but I couldn't. I tried everything. I cut calories and exercised like crazy, but the scale only went up. I thought I was making good food choices, but the food I was eating was actually slowing down my metabolism, without me even knowing it.

I dreaded being invited to a wedding or cocktail party, because it meant I would have to wear an unflattering dress. I avoided going anywhere that had a swimming pool. Buying the bathing suit cover-up became way more important than the bathing suit itself. I wouldn't allow anyone to see my body in a bikini. I never went into a pool or the ocean, I would just sit close to the water, covering the body that I had become so painfully ashamed of.

I FELT LIKE A SKINNY WOMAN TRAPPED IN AN OVERWEIGHT BODY

When it was my turn to have the Wine Country wedding of my dreams, I desperately tried to lose all of my unwanted body weight, but I wasn't able to exercise my way into the size wedding dress I wanted. My mother's words reverberated in my head: "you can't lose the weight after you turn 30!"

Then, I got pregnant with my first son. I gained 50 pounds during the pregnancy, which is significantly more weight than the doctors recommended. I spent the first 18 months of my son's life feeling ashamed of my body. I hated the body that gave life to my beautiful boy. My body had grown too big for me to love. I wish I could say that I found a way to love my body before losing the weight, but the truth is, I thought my body was betraying me and forcing me to be overweight, so I hated it. How can you love a body that you feel is betraying you?

I was sick of feeling like a thin woman but seeing a larger reflection every time I looked in the mirror. Out of this pain and desperation, I started trying new things and reading new books written by different doctors with totally different weight loss approaches. I had to re-learn everything I thought I knew about weight loss. Everything I learned during this time totally blew my mind.

IT IS NOT YOUR FAULT THAT YOU HAVEN'T LOST THE WEIGHT

The information is out there. It is very different than the weight loss advice that has been forced down our throats the past few decades, so it has not reached the mainstream yet, but I found countless doctors who were dying to get this information out. They were all saying the same thing, which is that 95% of all diets fail because diets lead to a predictable weight loss plateau, followed by inevitably regaining all of the weight back. They all showed clinical data proving that dieting slows down your metabolism.

This totally validated my experience. I want to validate for you too, that it is not your fault that you have not been able to lose the weight and keep it off. All of the weight loss advice that you have been told your entire life is hurting your metabolism and keeping you overweight.

What you are going to learn in this book is how to fix your broken metabolism and lose your unwanted weight. I will get to all of the juicy weight loss techniques shortly, I promise! Allow me to finish my story first; the story of how I joyfully found the secret to weight loss and proved my mama wrong.

SUCCESS IS NEVER A STRAIGHT LINE

I reluctantly tried the new weight loss techniques that I had learned from these doctors. I could not believe how quick and easy the pounds were flying off of my body! Not only did I finally lose all of my baby weight, but I also lost those additional 30 pounds that had been haunting me since my 30th birthday. I could not have been happier! I lost all of my weight in under six months, and once I hit my ideal weight, I got pregnant again.

I was elated to grow into a family of four, but in this state of elation, I went back to my old eating habits and gained 55 pounds! Quite frankly I indulged in way too many milkshakes to compensate for the fact that I couldn't drink wine! But thankfully, I had the tools under my belt and was able to shed all of the weight, once again. Since then, I have lost every unwanted pound and the scale has not gone up since.

I am proud to be at my ideal, healthy body weight and I am excited that I was able to do it after the age of 30 and after having birthed two big baby boys. I am proud that I effortlessly maintain my ideal body weight into my 40's. I am so happy to have proved my mother wrong.

Gone are the days of dreading being invited to a Wine Country wedding. Gone are the days of covering my body at the pool. I now proudly wear a bikini when I take my two sons to the swimming pool.

EXERCISE IS NOT THE PATH TO WEIGHT LOSS

Cutting calories and exercising did not help me lose weight. After several years of failing to lose weight, I was fortunate to have learned from the best doctors in the world that cutting calories and exercising do not lead to weight loss. These cutting-edge doctors taught me that eating certain foods makes it literally impossible to lose weight, no matter how much exercise you do.

WHAT YOU EAT & WHEN YOU EAT ARE CRITICAL TO WEIGHT LOSS

Once I learned what to eat and how to correctly time my meals, my constant sugar and carb cravings vanished. Now that I know what to eat and when to eat it, I easily maintain my ideal body weight and have the energy to keep up with my two active sons.

When I got my master's degree in psychology, I never dreamed that I would create a weight loss system to help other people lose weight. My own struggle to lose weight, however, became my soul calling. I am profoundly grateful for the opportunity to guide other people through a system that promotes both health and weight loss. My private clients have lost up to 75 pounds of unwanted body fat following the plan laid out for you in this book. I am excited to share every aspect of my proven weight loss system, known as the SEXY Diet, with you here. My vision is to inspire everyone to let their body and soul shine.

EVERYTHING IS POSSIBLE

Anybody can lose their unwanted body weight at any age, no matter what genes they inherited, no matter how many children they have had, no matter how much weight they have gained, no matter how many years they have lived in an overweight body. Anyone and everyone can have the body of their dreams at any age. No. Matter. What.

There is enormous pressure on the Western woman to be perfect. We are expected to be perfect mothers while being driven career women. We are supposed to be loving wives and good homemakers while maintaining an active social life. The media constantly bombards us with messages that tell us we need to be skinny, sexy, beautiful, funny, intelligent, successful and nice. We are made to feel that we are not meeting these expectations and that we are not good enough. Then we are inundated with images of other women on social media who appear to have it all, leaves us scrambling to meet an ideal that is impossible to achieve.

YOUR BODY WEIGHT IS NOT THE PROBLEM

You are not the problem; these constant messages are the problem. Embedded in the pages of this book, you will find the solution to this problem. You will not find messages in this book that will guilt trip you into being more sexy, skinny and beautiful. This book will not tell you that you are not sexy enough and that you need to quickly drop 40 pounds so that you will be sexier. This book will, however, teach you how to unleash the more confident, healthy, sexy version of yourself, that is, if you *want* to unleash the more confident, healthy, sexy version of yourself.

This book is going to be your go-to guide for everything that has to do with weight loss. Each chapter will teach you exactly what you need to do to shrink your fat cells, speed up your metabolism and activate your skinny genes. You will collect tools throughout this book that will completely transform your relationship with food. You will gain freedom from your sugar and carb addiction. You will move through guilt and shame and into a pleasurable relationship with eating. And most importantly, there are awesome practices and tools throughout this book that will catapult your self-esteem to heights you have never imagined.

Why go on another diet when you can go on a journey? The SEXY Diet is not a diet in the way that you are used to experiencing diets. You won't find yourself counting calories in and calories out. Ever. Rather, you are about to go on an epic journey. Your future-self is eternally grateful that you have decided to read this book and go on this soul nourishing journey. The future, sexier, healthier, happier version of yourself knows that this book holds the secrets that will transform you into the person you truly want to become.

HOW DO YOU KNOW IF YOU ARE SEXY?

Victoria's Secret does not define what it means to be sexy. Your age does not determine whether you can be sexy. Your body weight and size do not determine whether you are sexy. Your spouse or partner or former lovers do not get to determine whether you are sexy. Your mother, your friends, and your community do not decide whether you are sexy. And *I* certainly do not have a say in whether you are sexy. Sexy is not defined by how you look, how you act, or how others perceive you.

Sexy is a state of mind. Sexy is birthed out of confidence, liberty, health, inner beauty and authenticity. And the best part is, you get to define what sexy is for yourself. You will know, because you will *feel* it. When you unleash the more confident, healthier version of yourself, your inner, *sexy self* will have no choice but to come out and play.

UNLEASH THE SEXY BEAST WITHIN

The intention of this book is not to teach you how to be sexy, rather the intention is to empower you to reclaim the word, "sexy". Reclaim it from patriarchal objectification of the female body and reclaim it from the shame imposed on all women for not looking like a 22-year old lingerie model. The art of being sexy has nothing to do with looking a certain way or performing specific movements and behaviors. Reclaim the definition of sexy that was imposed on you and create the version of sexy that is authentic to you. What is your unique brand of sexy? Only you can answer that question.

Many of us have been conditioned to believe that it is sinful to express the sexier aspects of ourselves while others have been taught to overly sexualize their bodies in a way that does not feel safe or authentic. You need to reclaim the word, "sexy", so that you can discover and explore your authentically sexy nature. Reclaiming the word, "sexy" from the conditioning of your family and culture will elicit a transformation into a creative expression of your own unique sensuality. Sensuality is a natural part of being human; the authentic expression of your unique sensual nature allows you the freedom to unleash the sexy beast within.

YOU ARE GOD'S GREATEST GIFT

Experiencing a human life on this magnificent, blue planet is the highest honor and greatest gift given to you. You are a soul of great importance in the universe. You are a gorgeously unique expression of this creative energy we call God. There is no better expression of gratitude to your loving creator than by living your life to the fullest, continually moving toward your wildest dreams and living a truly connected, happy life.

YOU ARE SO MUCH MORE THAN JUST YOUR BODY

It is likely that you are reading this book to learn how to speed up your metabolism and lose weight. Yes, you will learn a simple and effective weight loss system that will lead to dramatic weight loss while speeding up your sluggish metabolism. People have lost over 75 pounds of unwanted body fat following this proven weight loss system. But weight loss is not the only benefit of the SEXY Diet. You will collect countless tools so that you will transform into the more confident, liberated, healthier and happier version of your current self. You are so much more than just your body; you will become intimately connected with your soul and learn how to let your soul shine.

Losing your unwanted body fat does not magically lead to self-confidence and a feeling of being sexy. The 4-part weight loss system, known as the SEXY Diet, focuses solely on the how to speed up your metabolism and burn off unwanted body fat. All of the other tools and practices contain the magic elixir you are looking for to unleash the more confident, healthier version of yourself.

EMOTIONAL WEIGHT LOSS

Getting to your ideal body weight will only get you part way to a more confident version of yourself. Each chapter contains proven techniques that will free you from the emotional weight you are carrying. Lose the stubborn pounds that have invaded your body and the stubborn thoughts that have invaded your mind. What unhealthy stories are you feeding your body? Do you consume unhealthy thoughts regularly, and do they consume you? Emotional weight is just as important to shed as physical weight.

You won't just lose weight when following the SEXY diet, you will also lose your fears of being seen by others in a bathing suit. You won't just gain a faster metabolism, you will also gain freedom from sugar and carb cravings. And I am thrilled to tell you that you will no longer be stuck with the genes you inherited that are keeping you in a heavier body. You are about to learn the secret of how to turn-on your skinny-genes! You are not stuck with a crappy genetic inheritance that will keep you overweight for life. You actually hit the gene-pool jack-pot, and I am going to tell you exactly how to find your genetic riches. Get ready to lose the emotional baggage you carry around and joyfully express your confident, healthier, thinner self.

Your inner wisdom already lies within. This book will help you move into a deeper relationship with your wise soul and place her in the driver's seat. Where would you rather be: comfortable with the status quo or free from cravings, free from body-shame, and liberated from unwanted body fat? Stop living in the past and create your amazing future!

TRANSFORM YOUR CONSCIOUSNESS

The SEXY diet is way more than just an eating plan. It is a lifestyle change. It will transform you. What transforms when you transform? Your body transformation is really just the icing on the cake; what really transforms is your consciousness. This is important because after reading this book, you will never go back to your old ways of eating with guilt, shame, and powerlessness. You will have a fast metabolism and an inner conviction that you are worthy of your new, healthier body. The SEXY diet will not teach you how to have discipline around food, rather, you will learn how to cultivate self-esteem and self-mastery in all areas of your life. Get ready to let your body and your soul shine!

CHAPTER 1

Do you Want the Salad or the Fries?

I remember going out to dinner with my father for his birthday, right around the time I had gained 30 unwanted pounds. My dad ordered salmon with vegetables for his birthday dinner, but as usual, I could not resist ordering the steak with french fries. While I waited for the main course to arrive, I compulsively ate a ton of bread with butter. I vividly remember sitting in that celebrated Napa Valley restaurant, stewing in shame, wondering, "when am I going to become the person who orders the healthy thing on the menu, rather than the thing that is going to keep me overweight?"

I wanted to be the kind of woman who ordered the salad instead of the fries. I wanted to choose the salad over the fries, not out of discipline, but from a place of desire. I wanted to *want* the salad instead of the fries, you know what I mean? I wanted to be able to say, "no, thank you" to dessert because I was too full for it anyway. But I didn't. I would always order the most epic chocolate dessert on the menu, and then feel uncomfortable, bloated and regretful after devouring it.

I used to finish every meal hating myself for always making bad decisions. You would have thought I had ordered a side of shame, a side of guilt and side of self-hatred with each meal.

EMPOWERMENT IS A CHOICE

While getting my master's degree in Psychology, I learned that you do not wake up one day and find that you have magically turned into the kind of person who chooses the salad over the french fries. You have to choose it. You have to choose to become an empowered person who makes empowering decisions. The empowered version of yourself is already living somewhere deep inside of you. You just have to choose to put him or her in the driver's seat. I have unleashed the thin woman that was living somewhere deep inside of my formerly overweight body. You can too. It is a choice.

I had to declare to myself that I am the kind of woman who orders the salad instead of the fries. I declared that I would unleash the thinner version of myself, and since I made this declaration several years ago, I now make empowered decisions every day. I am inspired to because it feels good. It is aligned with who I really am. You deserve to feel amazing in your body. You can! There is a power in declaring your goal. Declare what you want so that you can feel amazing in your body too!

WHO ARE YOU UNLEASHING?

What is your declaration? It is likely more than just weight loss. Do you want to be healthy? Do you want to be the kind of person who wakes up every morning and exercises or meditates? Do you want to quit your job and start your own business? Do you want to be the kind of person who eats salad for lunch every day? Do you want to be the kind of person who is irresistible and sexy in your skinny jeans? Who are you unleashing? There is a confident, healthier version of yourself trapped inside your body. Unleash the thinner you and let her shine.

HOW TO USE THIS BOOK

I want you to get the most out of this book by having a meaningful transformation. Of course, I want you to shed the pounds and regain your youthful energy. But I have other hopes for you as well. My prayerful intention for you is that you will have a transformation in how you engage with yourself. I want you to fall in love with yourself, because you are incredible and you are worthy of falling in love with.

When I was struggling with excess body weight, I did not feel like I was worthy of having someone fall in love with me. I didn't feel like I was worthy of much at all. I was at my heaviest at the time when I was interning as a clinical psychologist. I could not get the negative thoughts out of my head that told me that I had no right helping others because I had not figured out how to lose weight. I had a negative belief that constantly told me that there was something wrong with me because I couldn't lose the weight. I kept thinking that if there was something wrong with me, then how could I possibly help my clients make meaningful transformations in their lives? Wow, that's messed up, right? Well, actually, my training informs me that we all create stories like this in our heads, every day.

THE ONE THING HOLDING YOU BACK

I know that *you* likely carry stories about your weight in your head as well. These stories come from persistent, negative belief patterns and they are holding you back from your full potential. It is important for you to identify exactly how your excess body weight is holding you back so that you can intentionally become who you want to be.

How does your excess body weight affect your relationships? How is your weight affecting your job? How about your finances? Is your weight costing you money? You might be surprised by the answer when you dig deeper into that question! How is your weight affecting your self-esteem? Is it affecting your spiritual connection? How about your health? It is helpful to write these things down in a journal.

The false beliefs you hold and the story you are telling yourself about your excess body weight is likely way more damaging than your excess body weight itself. I know that was the case for me. In reality, I was making positive impacts on my clients, despite my excess body weight. In reality, you are a loveable, worthy, uniquely wonderful person, no matter what the scale says. The scale does not determine your self-worth. You are so worthy, just the way you are. And I applaud you for making this empowering decision to take charge of your health.

Your success in achieving your ideal body weight is largely going to be determined by your commitment to choose to be the healthier version of yourself right now, in this red-hot moment. Let's unleash the healthier, thinner, sexier version of yourself now.

CHAPTER 2

How to Fix a Broken Metabolism

WOULD YOU GIVE DOG FOOD TO A LION?

I have some very bad news for you. You are an animal. I know, I know, we humans tend to think of ourselves as being superior to animals. We typically classify every creature, other than humans, as animals. But the hard truth is, we humans are nothing more than animals with remarkable brains and opposable thumbs.

When you go to a zoo, you get to observe animals out of their natural habitat. They don't always do the best job given their limited space, but zoo's really go to painstaking efforts to mimic the natural habitat of each of the animals, so that the animals don't die. If you have ever been to a lion exhibit during feeding time, you will see that they feed the lions the same kind of food that the lions would hunt for as if they were roaming the African tundra. They do not feed dog food to the lions.

The same goes for the elephants, gorillas and sea otters. Zoos across the world diligently feed every animal exactly what that animal it is supposed to eat, as if it were still living in the wild. They never throw in a handful of kibble to the elephants, just because kibble might taste good to an elephant.

Here's the thing, ladies. We humans are not eating anything close to what was formerly eaten in our "natural habitat". The standard American diet is the equivalent of taking a lion, putting it in a cage fit for a kitten, and offering it dog food. A feline carnivore, such as a lion, should only eat the flesh of another animal that it hunted, not kibble.

I am not saying that humans need to go back to the hunter and gatherer days, but we do need to start eating something that is similar to what our ancestors ate. I am not talking about the Paleo diet, rather we need to start including more food that is actually *real* food. What I am really saying is, OMG, stop feeding yourself dog food! Your body is not meant to survive on cereal bars, crackers, non-fat vanilla lattes, sodas and frozen dinners! These processed foods are like dog food for your body. I am not kidding you! You are not supposed to eat that crap. Candy is kibble, not human food. Fast food is kibble, not human food. Chips are kibble, not human food. I am begging you, please, have some self-respect and stop treating yourself like a dog. Stop feeding yourself kibble! You deserve way better than that! OK, I'm sorry I was so harsh about this, but honestly, I am so glad I got that off of my chest.

YOU ARE A SEXY BEAST

My point is, you are not a dog, so stop feeding yourself kibble. You *are* a sexy beast! So, what does a sexy beast eat? The four components of the SEXY diet is exactly what a sexy beast eats. SEXY is actually

17

just a fun acronym I use so people can easily remember my proven 4-part weight loss system. The SEXY diet is all about speeding up your metabolism, turning on your skinny genes and burning off all of your unwanted, unneeded body fat. And no, you will not be asked to eat kibble when following the SEXY diet. There are four simple and effective steps of the proven weight loss system, known as the SEXY diet.

THE SEXY DIET DEFINED

The **S** stands for Sugar & Flour Free
The **E** stands for Eat an Abundance of Vegetables
The **X** stands for eXtend your Period of Fasting
The **Y** stands for Yes to Healthy Fats

And that is the recipe for **SEXY**.

I FIXED MY BROKEN METABOLISM AND YOU CAN TOO

My weight loss journey was excruciating. It took years of yo-yo dieting before I discovered how to fix my broken metabolism and return to my ideal body weight. I do not want anyone else to ever have to go through the pain and struggle I went through. That said, there is always gleaming treasure buried deep beneath our pain, which was certainly the case for me. I am grateful for the years of hardship I endured because out of this emotional pain, I birthed a conviction to help others. My frustration and despair became my inspiration to create this effective 4-part weight loss system called the SEXY Diet that has transformed the lives and bodies of countless others.

It is said that when someone makes a positive impact on another person's life, it creates an exponential ripple effect of positivity. This really excites me because together, you and I are going to elicit positive transformations in countless others. When you start seeing results by following the SEXY Diet, you are likely going to tell a minimum of five other people about it. When each of those five people start seeing positive results, they will each tell five other people and on and on. It is impossible to know how many lives will be impacted; what *is* known is that positivity breeds more positivity and I am humbled at the opportunity to positively transform countless lives, with you as my co-creator. Let's do this! It all begins with your amazing transformation. You are going to love exploring all of the delicious details of the SEXY diet and begin your smokin' hot transformation.

CHAPTER 3

The S in SEXY

IS YOUR BREAKFAST MAKING YOU FAT?

I gained my excess 30 pounds over a decade ago and the outdated nutrition advice we were given back then was to never skip meals and to always eat breakfast. It was then believed that breakfast would somehow rev up your metabolism, so I dutifully ate my bowl of granola every single morning. I bought the granola at the health food store, so I assumed it was healthy.

The problem is, I could never make it to lunch without being ravenously hungry. I assumed that I was hungry because I wasn't eating enough. Soon, my ¾ cup portion, the suggested serving size, doubled. At first, I would get very full off of my 1 & ½ cup serving of granola with milk. But after a while, I noticed that, once again, I was ravenously hungry an hour before lunch. I kept wondering, "what is wrong with me that I cannot go three flippin' hours without stuffing food in my face?" I now know the answer to that embarrassing question. Before I answer it, let's dig a little deeper into the calories of my breakfast of choice.

NOT ALL CALORIES ARE CREATED EQUAL

When you have weight you want to lose, the first thing that probably comes to your mind is that you are going to have to eat less calories and exercise more. It has become my mission in life to inform people that this is not true. The most common weight loss plan that we have all been brainwashed to believe, "eat less calories and exercise more", has failed us because it has failed to understand the most important thing about calories: not all calories are created equal. A 250-calorie candy bar does not do the same thing to your body as 250-calories of vegetables. You intuitively know that, but at the same time you have been told a million times that all calories are created equal and if you just cut calories, then you will lose weight.

This is a rotten lie and your metabolism has been damaged because of this lie. Most people do not lose weight when they cut calories, because hormones play a big role in the weight loss game. Certain foods trigger certain hormones, which greatly impact your body's ability gain and lose weight.

SPRAYING MIRACLE-GRO ON YOUR FAT CELLS

Sugar and processed flour are a special category of food because they both trigger the hormone *insulin*. Insulin dramatically impacts whether you can burn fat. Insulin is known as the blood sugar hormone, but it is also the *fat-storing* hormone. Insulin is like Miracle-Gro for your fat cells. It literally tells your fat cells to grab all of the calories it can find and hoard them.

Insulin forces the calories you eat into your fat cells, making your fat cells grow bigger and bigger. Every time you eat sugar or processed foods, like granola and, you know, *kibble*, you are spraying Miracle-Gro on your fat cells.

This brings us to the S in SEXY. The SEXY Diet begins with the letter S, which stands for, "sugar & flour free." The very first step of the SEXY Diet is to remove the empty calorie, processed foods from your diet, such as granola, so you can replace those calories with a healthier alternative. There are virtually no nutrients in sugar and processed flour. These two ingredients are an unnecessary waste of calories. But more importantly, eating foods laced with sugar and refined flour slow down your metabolism. That is not sexy!

Why does successful weight loss begin with ditching sugar and flour? Because they increase your insulin levels more than any other food. Every time you eat sugar, you are spraying Miracle-Gro on your fat cells. Every time you eat pasta, candy, bread, crackers, or gluten-free cookies, you are spraying Miracle-Gro on your fat cells and slowing down your metabolism.

My daily bowl of granola was the Miracle-Gro I was spraying on my fat cells. It was literally making me gain weight and preventing me from burning fat when I exercised. You are probably wondering if you can just exercise all that kibble and Miracle-Gro away. When your insulin levels are high after you eat these foods, you cannot exercise your fat away. If you are restricting your calories, but still including lots of sugar and flour, your body will respond by slowing down your metabolism. I have never exercised as much in my life as I did during the time I was at my heaviest. It wasn't the amount of calories that I was eating that was making me gain weight; my food choices were making it impossible to lose the weight. Is this starting to make sense?

Why I Couldn't Go 3 Flippin' Hours Without Stuffing Food in my Face

Have you ever eaten a huge breakfast, only to find yourself ravenously hungry before your lunch break? This happens to a lot of people and is way more common than you would think. It's not *you*, it's the food you ate for breakfast. I used to feel so ashamed of myself for always being hungry. I know *now* that I was unable to discern between true hunger and hunger that was triggered by hormones running amuck from foods laced with sugar and refined flour. I know *now* that sugar and flour were putting me in a constant state of hunger. I thought I was a bad person for always being hungry and for often failing to fight the urge to snack between meals. My hunger was real, but I did not need the food for nutrients. My hunger was triggered by out-of-whack hormones.

Granola was once considered a health food, but in reality, it is a processed food, full of refined sugar and processed flour, foods I lump in a category that I affectionately call, "kibble". Like most processed foods, granola slows down your metabolism, storing excess body fat, and making you hungry for no good reason.

For successful weight loss, sugar and flour have got to go. You can reverse the damage to your metabolism immediately by cutting out these foods and replacing them with a healthier alternative. Knowledge is power! Now you know the biggest offenders in your diet and you can immediately begin to speed up your metabolism by reducing them. Reducing my sugar and flour intake has dramatically changed my life. What foods are you eating that are acting like Miracle-Gro for your fat cells? Remove these foods from your diet so that you can lose all of your unwanted body fat today! Let's continue on our SEXY journey, shall we?

CHAPTER 4

The E in SEXY

TURN ON YOUR SKINNY GENES

No book about weight loss is complete without a section devoted to your genes. I am not talking about the blue jeans that you wear, but rather the genes you were born with, you know, the stuff that contains your DNA. I have countless clients tell me that they were born with terrible, horrible, no good genes that force them to live in a heavier body. I love proving them wrong! The reason why they are wrong to believe that they are unlucky in the genetics department is because genes do not work the way most people think they do.

Most people believe that they were born with specific genes and that they are stuck with those specific genes for life. For instance, if you were born with blue eyes, then you inherited the blue-eyed gene. If you have brown eyes, then you got the brown-eyed gene. But not all genes work that way. It *is* true that you are stuck with the genes you were born with, *but* you were born with a lot more genes than the ones you are currently using!

Look at it this way, if you were unlucky enough to have been born with the gene that predisposes you to breast cancer, there is not one doctor in the world who would tell you that you will definitely get breast cancer. Just because you have a gene, doesn't mean that the gene will turn on and give you cancer. Are you following me? I have some awesome news for you! There is a phenomenon called genetic expression, which means you can turn a gene *on* or turn a gene *off*. Your best bet is to do everything in your power to turn off the dreaded breast cancer gene.

The brilliant, triple board-certified physician, Dr. Zach Bush, says that from your genes, you can make four million different bodies. If you don't like the body you are living in right now, don't freak out! There are literally four million other bodies that you can have! FOUR MILLION! You can change your body right now to one that you *do* like. Dr. Bush says that nutrition is the number one way that you are going to be able to change your body. What you put in your mouth today is literally who you become. Your food shapes your metabolism, your thoughts, your mind, your body weight, your health, and every other aspect of what kind of body you have. How cool is that? You have options. You have power!

The reason that all of my clients who say they were born with the "slow metabolism gene" are dead wrong, is because we were *all* born with the slow metabolism gene. We were also all born with the fast metabolism gene. It's all about how to turn off the slow metabolism gene and how to turn on your skinny genes. Raise your hand if you want to turn on your skinny genes!

How do you turn on your skinny genes and have a fast metabolism? It's easy. You can turn on your skinny genes by eating certain foods. It really is *that* simple! There are these crazy-smart scientists over in the UK studying this phenomenon right now and they have discovered that a certain kind of antioxidant called *polyphenols* will turn on your skinny genes. There are thousands of different kinds of polyphenols and the more of them we eat in a wide variety, the better.

THE BLUE ZONES

Have you heard of the blue zones? The blue zones are the five areas in the world where more people live to be 100 than anywhere else in the world. The five blue zones are Loma Linda, California, Sardinia, Italy, Okinawa, Japan, Nicoya, Costa Rica, and Icaria, Greece. The 100-year-olds living in these five blue zones are running around like healthy 60-year-olds. Everyone living in the blue zones appear to be healthier, thinner, and fitter than anywhere else in the world.

Thousands of scientists have flocked to these blue zones, studying everything about them, in hopes of discovering the fountain of youth. It turns out that the one thing they all have in common is that the healthy people living in all five of the blue zones are eating a diet rich in polyphenols. And get this: when people living in the blue zones move, and start eating a different diet, they stop living to be 100. In fact, in a very short period of time, people who change their diet from one that is high in polyphenols, to a standard American diet, well, they get sick and gain weight, like clockwork.

Those crazy-smart scientists in the UK have done some studies on people who don't live in blue zones but eat like someone who does. It turns out that just by increasing the amount of polyphenols in your diet, you can turn on your skinny genes, lose weight, decrease inflammation, and improve your overall health. These scientists have found eight specific skinny genes that you can turn on, just by eating a diet that includes lots of polyphenols every day.

WHAT DOESN'T KILL YOU MAKES YOU STRONGER

You know that Kelly Clarkson song, "What Doesn't Kill You Makes You Stronger"? Polyphenols work *that* way. They are actually a little bit stressful for your body, but in a really good way. Let me explain.

When you exercise, you are putting a little bit of stress on your body. A little bit of stress is a good thing because it makes you stronger. The same thing happens when you take a cold shower, spend time in a hot sauna, or practice intermittent fasting. All of these things put a little bit of stress on your body. A little bit of stress on your body turns on certain genes and hormonal responses that make you healthier. Polyphenols do the same thing. Polyphenols are found in certain vegetables, fruits, herbs and spices. Every time you eat them, your body gives off a stress alarm. This stress signal turns on the genes that make you stronger to protect you from future stress. But it turns out, these stress signals also make you *skinnier*. They literally turn on your skinny genes. Literally!

ARE YOU READY FOR SOME GOOD NEWS?

Polyphenols also make your skin glow. Do you want more radiant skin? Of course, you do!

ARE YOU READY FOR SOME MORE GOOD NEWS?

You are probably already eating polyphenols every day. If you want to turn on your skinny genes, you just need to eat more of them. You can do this by replacing some of your unhealthier meals with more polyphenols.

ARE YOU READY FOR SOME EVEN MORE GOOD NEWS?

You can eat more polyphenols by having a super yummy lunch every day. The best way to do this is to eat a big, fat salad for lunch. I am passionate about teaching my clients the art of making vegetables taste amazing. My clients love my signature, *Fat Salad*! This is my favorite way to make veggies so delicious that I actually crave them!

THE FAT SALAD THAT MAKES YOU SKINNY

My signature *Fat Salad* is super easy and OMG delicious. Here is exactly how to make my super yummy *Fat Salad* to turn on your skinny genes: Instead of iceberg lettuce, choose arugula, spinach, and red endive. These lettuces are super high in polyphenols. The best polyphenol rich vegetables to throw in each of your salads are: red onions, celery, radishes of every color, asparagus, olives, capers, ¼ cup berries, ½ ounce of pecans, one tablespoon of pumpkin seeds, extra virgin olive oil and the juice of ½ lemon. Also add some fresh or dried herbs, because herbs and spices are loaded with polyphenols. I love adding either thyme, dill or cilantro to my salads, choose whatever tastes best to you. Ultimately, you want to diversify the foods you eat so that you will get lots of different polyphenols, so choose differently every time and always eat the rainbow. Lastly, add salt and pepper and your taste buds will be as happy as your metabolism. I always eat avocado with my salad for the extra fat and nutrients, but I wait to cut it open until I am ready to eat my salad if I make my salad in advance. You can make up to five of these salads on a lazy Sunday evening, so that you can blast your body with polyphenols each day of your work week!

The crazy-smart scientists have found that adding protein to your polyphenol rich meals helps digest the polyphenols even more, so add either two hardboiled eggs, two slices of bacon, or three ounces of chicken to your salad. If you are a vegetarian, stick with nuts and seeds. Flax seed is rich in polyphenols, so add some flax and more pumpkin seeds or sunflower seeds to your salad!

BONUS CHEAT

Here is a bonus polyphenol rich food: Chocolate. Raise your hand if you love chocolate! If you need a snack mid-day, go for an ounce or two of chocolate with some almonds or walnuts. But ditch the Hershey's. They kill all the polyphenols and add a ton of metabolism slowing sugar. You need to find chocolate from one of the many companies who preserve the polyphenol content of the chocolate. Look for chocolate bars with a 78% or higher cacao content. Ideally it will be sweetened with xylitol or stevia, not cane sugar or high fructose corn syrup. Look for chocolate that is low in sugar and high in cacao. This is my favorite cheat because it tastes amazing without slowing down your metabolism. Enjoy your polyphenol rich foods to turn on your skinny genes so you can easily slip into your skinny jeans.

THE E IN SEXY STANDS FOR, "EAT AN ABUNDANCE OF VEGETABLES"

Not everybody thinks that vegetables are SEXY, but hear me out. The FDA recommends that we eat somewhere between 5-9 servings of fruits and vegetables every day. It is estimated that far less than 15% of American's come even close to that. We need to do better, my friends. We need to eat more vegetables.

Instead of eating nutrient dense vegetables, most Americans are consuming far too many processed foods, which are devoid of nutrients. Processed foods are high in calories and are like Miracle-Gro for your fat cells. We need to replace our processed foods with nutrient dense foods, such as vegetables. Vegetables do not slow down your metabolism. Vegetables do not make your fat cells grow. Vegetables turn on your skinny genes so you can eat as many of them as your magnificent heart desires!

Vegetables should be the foundation of each meal. We have been conditioned to think of veggies as a side dish. From now on, I want you to load up your plate with veggies. At least half of your meal, in volume, should consist of vegetables. At least half! My dinners are usually 2/3 vegetables. Vegetables give you the vitamins, minerals, and fiber you need for healthy weight loss. Mix it up. Eat salads, fermented vegetables and steamed veggies. Go for green veggies and avoid starchy vegetables such as potatoes and corn. And no, ketchup is not a vegetable, no matter what the government says! Include lots of green leafy vegetables. Try to include more than one vegetable with each meal; diversity of vegetables is important for your health. Including more vegetables in your diet is how you are going to turn on your skinny genes so you can slip into your sexy skinny jeans!

WHY CHOOSE ORGANIC?

It is common knowledge that you are not supposed to mix bleach and ammonia. Combining bleach and ammonia will instantly release toxic vapors resulting in illness ranging from nausea and vomiting, to temporary loss of vision, and in extreme cases can be fatal. The tale of two common household products, that can become fatal when combined, illustrates the potential hidden dangers of all chemicals, when combined.

There are over 80,000 chemicals lurking everywhere. These chemicals are in your food, your bed, your furniture, your electronics, your car, your clothes, your beauty and skin care products, and even your medicines and vaccines. It blows my mind that only a tiny fraction of the chemicals we are exposed to daily have been tested for safety. Not only are most chemicals not tested for safety, but then imagine what happens when you start combining these chemicals. Maybe one chemical is generally safe, but if you combine it with another chemical, it might have a similar reaction to that of bleach and ammonia when combined.

The truth is, we have no idea what happens when we are exposed to multiple chemicals. Nobody does. Not the EPA, not your doctor, not your mom, and not the companies who are producing these chemicals. Sadly, we will likely never know. There is no independent testing because the tools to test whether any of these chemicals harm us *do not exist*. Let that sink in. While a few chemicals have been tested for safety, the vast majority of the 80,000 chemicals we are exposed to have no tests to prove their safety.

I think about the poor housewife who learned the hard way about mixing ammonia and bleach. It wasn't always common knowledge that these two chemicals react in such a harmful way. How many people made the mistake of mixing these two powerful chemicals while innocently cleaning their homes? How many of us are innocently being harmed by a mixture of two or more chemicals that we are unknowingly being exposed to?

It enrages me when somebody claims that chemicals are safe because the government allows them. After I try my best not to flip this person off, I respond by compassionately telling them that the government doesn't have the tools to measure whether any of the chemicals we are being exposed to daily are safe. Our government has chosen to trust the very industries that are profiting from producing these chemicals. Would you trust someone, who is making millions of dollars off of a product, to tell you whether that product is safe? They have no financial incentive to test for safety, so why would they?

It is true that some chemicals have been tested for safety and have earned the classification, GRAS, which means that are "generally recognized as safe". However, two chemicals that are *generally recognized as safe* have never been tested together. Never. It has never been done! The scary thing is, we are never only exposed to one chemical. We are exposed to dozens if not hundreds of chemicals every single day. For example, conventional strawberries are sprayed with a totally different herbicide than conventional wheat, which is sprayed with a totally different chemical than sugar is sprayed with. Conventional dairy contains several different chemicals than all the rest. Put all of these chemicals together and you will find a strawberry shortcake teeming with over a dozen different pesticides, herbicides and chemicals, some of which may have been tested in isolation, but *never* together. Nobody knows how all of those chemicals might react together. How messed up is that?

The reason why I am so passionately angry about this topic is because I am a mom of two young boys. Even if a handful of the 80,000 chemicals we are exposed to *have* been tested and are generally regarded as safe, *children* and their sensitive immune systems have never been tested. Clinical studies show that there is no level of pesticides that is safe for children. These studies also inform us that even a small amount of pesticides can do a significant amount of harm to some children.

The other reason why I am so passionately angry about this topic is because I am a daughter of two dead parents. Nobody knows why my parents both got cancer and nobody will ever know why both of my parents died as a result of their cancer before their 60ᵗʰ birthdays. What I do know is that I live in an agricultural area, where herbicides and pesticides are sprayed in abundance. These chemicals are in the water my family bathes in and in the air we breathe. My mother's cancer diagnosis came at the age of 41, which is ridiculously young. My father regularly sprayed these chemical herbicides and pesticides on the grapes that he grew. We will never know if these chemicals contributed to the cancer that took the lives of my parents, but I do know that I am going to do everything in my power to protect my body and my children's bodies. I do this by choosing organic food whenever possible.

I passionately urge you to consider organic. Please think about the farmers, their families, your children, the air we all breathe and the water we all bathe in when making this decision. Yes, organic is often more expensive, but it reduces your overall toxic load and studies show that organic foods contain a significantly higher level of nutrients, including polyphenols. Remember, polyphenols are the antioxidant that literally turn your skinny genes on. If organic isn't your thing, but weight loss is, then choosing organic is going to get you to your ideal weight way faster. So, maybe organic really is your thing, after all!

CHAPTER 5

The X in SEXY

CIRCADIAN RHYTHM

You are probably familiar with the term *circadian rhythm*. It is not usually considered a sexy topic, but there are actually some super sexy things about your circadian rhythm, so let's dive in a little deeper, shall we? For those who don't know, your circadian rhythm is your body's internal clock that keeps you on a 24-hour cycle. It is why you are naturally inclined to sleep at night and awaken with the sun. It was previously believed that sunlight affects your circadian rhythm the most, but it turns out that *food* also has a huge impact on your circadian rhythm. It's not so much *what* you eat, but *when* you eat that affects your circadian rhythm.

And guess what? Ten years of clinical research tells us that *when* you eat profoundly affects your weight as well. This is mind blowing stuff, because they didn't just do this research once or twice. They have done it hundreds of times and the outcome always shows that *when* you eat is just as important as *what* you eat.

NOT ALL CALORIES ARE CREATED EQUAL, REVISITED

Clinical studies always seem to begin in a lab with mice, and these studies are no exception. It began when they fed two sets of mice the same crappy diet of high-fat and high-sugar foods. They fed both sets of mice the exact same number of calories but one set of mice had to eat all of their food in just an eight-hour window, while the other set of mice was allowed to eat their food whenever they wanted. The mice who ate during the eight-hour window had no weight gain on their crappy diet while the other mice all gained a significant amount of weight. Remember, they ate the same number of calories!

How is it possible that mice who ate the same number of calories had a totally different outcome? It is because calories are not nearly as important as we have all been brainwashed to believe. They have done this experiment over and over with the same results. Not only did the mice who ate all of their food in an eight-hour window not gain weight, but they also had normal cholesterol levels, normal insulin levels, and pretty much all of their major health markers were totally better than the mice who ate whenever they wanted.

They have also tested this on humans in a controlled clinical setting, and guess what? The humans who ate whatever they wanted over a nine-hour eating window had the same outcome as the mice. These people did not eat crazy amounts of junk food, they were just instructed to eat whatever they would normally eat, but nothing was allowed to go in their mouths outside of their nine-hour eating window, not even a single blueberry!

After 16-weeks, nobody had gained any weight and they all reported sleeping better. Hello, circadian rhythms! There is more exciting information about circadian rhythms, but before we get to that, I have to tell you my favorite part of this clinical study. All of the people who ate during the nine-hour eating window reported feeling less hunger. Who wants to feel less hunger? Pretty much everyone!

We have all been brainwashed to believe that we need to count calories in order to lose weight. Calories really are not that important. What *is* important is choosing the *right* calories and knowing when to eat those calories. These experiments have told us so much. We now know that our human bodies need at least 14-hours a day where we are not eating, so our body gets a break from the super hard work of digestion.

YOUR EATING WINDOW

Ideally, you should eat in a six to eight-hour window most days, such as from 10am-6pm or Noon-6pm. It is also best to give your body at least three hours after eating your last meal before going to bed. So always aim to eat an early dinner. And remember, you cannot have any food after your eating window has closed, not even a single blueberry!

HOW CIRCADIAN RHYTHMS TURN ON OUR SKINNY GENES

The scientists have proved that your very first meal of the day sets your circadian rhythm the same way that sunlight does. Your first bite of the day tells your metabolism to do its job. That's the good news. The bad news is that if you keep eating all day and into the night, it confuses your circadian rhythm and your body thinks it is still day time when it is night time because it is still digesting. Your body responds to a longer circadian rhythm cycle by storing more fat and giving you a crappy night's sleep. That is not sexy. The take-away from this is to eat in a shorter window of time so that you will have a faster metabolism and lose more weight with ease.

There is still much more research to be done in this area, but these studies are very exciting. When you eat at the same time every day, and more importantly, stop eating in the early evening, you are telling your body when it is daytime and when it is nighttime. Who doesn't want to sleep better and be thinner?

Your eating window begins as soon as you take a sip of your morning coffee, unless your coffee is black. Cream and sugar start your feeding window. If you have a small snack before bedtime, even if it is just a little bit of honey in your tea, a nibble of a cookie, or a single blueberry, your window does not close until those very last calories have been swallowed. You must make sure that your last bite of dinner is your last bite of the day so that you will sleep better, be thinner, and healthier.

WEIGHT LOSS VS. WEIGHT MAINTENANCE

The strategy of eating in a time-restricted window of time is a game changer because you will not gain weight when you eat this way. This is not a weight *loss* plan though, it is a weight *maintenance* plan. If you want to maintain your weight, look no further than this time-restricted eating plan. It is the best strategy for you to maintain your ideal body weight, once you reach your ideal body weight.

If you want to *lose* weight, there are a few extra steps to take in conjunction with this time-restricted eating plan. I will detail other methods of fasting so you can learn the best method for weight loss in the chapter entitled, "Burn Off the Calories You Overate Last Month, Today".

CHAPTER 6

The Y in SEXY

FAT DOES NOT MAKE YOU FAT

We have all been brainwashed to believe that fat makes you fat. This is a filthy lie. Fat does not make you fat! Sugar makes you fat. Processed carbohydrates make you fat. Fat makes you *lean*. That said, there are *good* fats and there are *bad* fats and it is important that you know the difference because the bad fats can contribute to weight gain.

UNHEALTHY FATS

Everyone knows that fried foods and trans fats are really really bad for you. But most people are surprised to learn that vegetable oils that are high in polyunsaturated fat are also unhealthy. Polyunsaturated vegetable oils lead to weight gain because they cause inflammation. When following the SEXY diet, do not include polyunsaturated vegetable oils.

We have been told for decades that polyunsaturated vegetable oils, such as canola oil, sunflower oil, safflower oil, corn oil and soybean oil are healthy oils, when eaten in moderation. These refined, processed vegetable oils have been mistakenly believed to be safer alternatives because they come from a vegetable. Sadly, they are wreaking havoc on your health.

In a nutshell, polyunsaturated fat is not bad in and of itself. But processing, refining and heating polyunsaturated fat is bad because these fats oxidize very easily under these conditions. What happens when they oxidize is they create free-radicals. Free-radicals can be very dangerous for your health, causing inflammation and potentially a host of other health problems. Polyunsaturated fats, even in moderation, are very bad for you and need to be eliminated so that you can maximize your weight loss potential.

HEALTHY FATS

I have read so many books written by different doctors and sifted through countless clinical studies. I have absolute confidence that extra virgin olive oil, when used at room temperature or slightly warmed, is a health food. I have confidence that coconut oil is a health food. I have confidence that butter, sourced from grass-fed cows, is a health food.

Healthy fats not only fill you up, but they are great for your brain health, make your skin glow, speed up your metabolism, and transform vegetables from boring to delicious. I encourage you to lightly steam your broccoli and put as much grass-fed butter on it as you want. Steamed broccoli and kale with grass-fed butter is one of my favorite things to eat with dinner. Enjoy your vegetables with healthy fats. Your brain and metabolism will love you for it!

I'M TOTALLY NUTS

I rarely go a day without eating a few raw nuts or seeds. Nuts and seeds are nutrient dense foods, containing loads of vitamins and minerals that are missing from most diets. They are a wonderful source of healthy fat and protein. They give you the feeling of satiety and are wonderful additions to salads, smoothies or a bento-box style meal. I like to use hydrated chia seeds as the base for my smoothies. I also occasionally add flax seeds for healthy fat and fiber.

Since we are on the topic of smoothies, I will take this opportunity to remind you that smoothies should be very low in sugar, even if the sugar is coming from natural sources, such as fruit. Basically, if it tastes like dessert, then it *is* dessert and should not be considered a health food because it has Miracle-Gro in it. You can totally add fruit to your smoothie to make it taste good, but choose berries and never use more than one cup of berries in each smoothie. Also, if you are going to drink smoothies, drink them slowly. I like to chew my smoothies, which sounds weird, but chewing is an important part of digestion. Ideally you chew while sipping so that you properly digest your smoothie.

OK, back to nuts and seeds. A small handful of sprouted pumpkin seeds or sunflower seeds, followed by a large glass of water can be an incredibly filling, nutrient dense snack that can guard against cravings, give you energy, and prevent you from overeating unhealthy foods!

My favorite healthy fats that I include in my diet nearly every day are avocados, olives, macadamia nuts, pumpkin seeds, coconut oil, MCT oil, which is a derivative of coconut oil, and extra virgin olive oil.

HIDDEN DANGERS LURKING IN YOUR OLIVE OIL

A word of caution about extra virgin olive oil: the vast majority of extra virgin olive oil that has been tested in the U.S. is not really extra virgin olive oil. It is frequently diluted with unhealthy, cheap fats, such as canola oil. When buying extra virgin olive oil, make sure you are buying independently tested, lab-certified extra virgin olive oil so that you can ensure pureness. I never buy extra virgin olive oil from Italy. Never. As much as I love Italy and dream of returning there daily, the Italian extra virgin olive oil industry has sadly been taken over by the Italian Mafia. I wish this was a joke, but it isn't. Italian olive oils have been reported to have the highest levels of being diluted with cheaper oils. To make matters worse, they also ship the olive oil to the U.S. on cargo ships, which have a long transit time. Freshness is important when it comes to extra virgin olive oil, so it is best to pass on Italian olive oils.

I am extremely lucky to live in the Northern California Wine Country because so many wineries also produce their own extra virgin olive oil. I frequently buy it fresh from one of my favorite organic wineries. Other times I find local, organic extra virgin olive oil at the farmers market. These are the best options when buying extra virgin olive oil.

The last important detail about extra virgin olive oil is that it does not like to be heated. It starts producing those yucky free-radicals when it gets too hot, so it is best to use it on salads or to drizzle on foods after they have been cooked. Use coconut oil and grass-fed butter when cooking at higher temperatures!

A MATCH MADE IN HEAVEN

Some people don't love the E in SEXY, which is, "Eat an Abundance of Vegetables". What I love about the Y in SEXY, which is "Yes to Healthy Fats", is that you get to drizzle as much fat on your veggies as you want to make them taste amazing! Veggies and fat are a match made in heaven. Fat makes everything taste better, especially veggies.

Here are my favorite ways to enjoy my veggies: I always drizzle a tablespoon of local, fresh extra virgin olive oil on my salads. I also steam veggies for dinner and either dress them with as much grass-fed butter or coconut oil as I want. Adding spices to my steamed vegetables also give them an explosion of flavor with the added benefit of polyphenols! I love adding butter and coriander to my steamed squash and kale. Roasted butternut squash with coconut oil and Ceylon cinnamon is life-changing. Steamed broccoli with garlic butter is mouthwatering. You are going to start loving your veggies once you start experimenting with healthy fats. Do not be scared of adding too much fat!

HOW TO NOT FEEL HUNGRY ALL THE TIME

If you live on planet earth, then you have been told over and over again that dietary fat is unhealthy and that it will make you gain weight. It is likely going to take you some time to re-program your brain to associate eating *fat* with weight loss. Please take the time to re-program this horrible lie that *fat makes you fat*, because restricting fat has damaged your metabolism. Healthy fats are awesome. Fat has an amazing hormonal effect on your body: it actually turns your hunger hormones *off* and turns the hormones that make you feel full *on*. Fat makes you *full*, not *fat*! It is not the volume of food in your belly that makes you feel full, it's the kind of food you are eating that gives you the feeling of lasting satiety. Fat is king when it comes to making you feel full after a meal. Healthy fats not only taste great, but they are also the opposite of Miracle-Gro for your fat cells! Eating healthy fats daily are way more important to me than taking vitamins.

SAY YES TO HEALTHY FAT AT EVERY MEAL TO:

1. Speed up your metabolism
2. Make your vegetables taste amazing
3. Feel full for several hours after every meal
4. Give your brain a boost
5. Make your skin glow

CHAPTER 7

Your Success Story Begins Now

TOOL BOX OF SUCCESSFUL WEIGHT LOSS

I am going to give you a tool box now, albeit an imaginary one, and throughout the rest of the book, I will keep giving you tools to put inside your SEXY new tool box. By the end of this book, you will have tons of incredible power tools that are going to help you become the healthiest, thinnest version of yourself. Use these tools to sculpt and chisel the body of your dreams. Open up your tool box and put in the following new, shiny tools!

The 4-steps of the SEXY diet have already been placed in your tool box of successful weight loss. Think of these four tools as your *Master Tools*. They must be used regularly in order for you to achieve your ideal body weight. We will explore them deeper in the following chapters so that they can easily be integrated into your life. We will also add many more fun power tools for you to use on your weight loss journey. Let's begin collecting more tools, shall we?

YOUR FUTURE SELF

One of my favorite tools that is sitting in your shiny new tool box of successful weight loss is *visualization*. How does this tool, called visualization, work for weight loss? I promise, you will unleash the thinner version of yourself when you use the tool of visualization every day. Specifically, I want you to visualize, in your mind's eye, your *future self*. This future self is the version of yourself who has achieved your ideal body weight and has dramatically improved her health.

Your future, success-story version of yourself is sexy, healthy, energetic and amazing, that is, if you want your future self to be sexy, healthy, energetic and amazing. It is totally up to you. You get to create your future, success-story version of yourself. You do this by imagining what your goals, hopes and dreams are. Visualization is going to become one of your most cherished tools. It is a foundational tool and is absolutely critical for your success.

VISUALIZATION IN ACTION

When Taylor Swift was a child, she would imagine what it would be like to receive a Grammy award and literally give an acceptance speech in the mirror, while holding a hair brush as if it was her microphone. She visualized her success at a young age, over and over again, and literally created her reality. Nearly all Olympic athletes spend time every day visualizing each race. They *feel* into what it will be like, look like, smell like, and sound like every step of the way. They imagine the results they want, every single day. This tool of visualization is what gives elite athletes an edge over the rest.

You must use the tool of visualization to create the future of your dreams so that all of your dreams will come true. Get a clear image in your mind's eye of what you want to look like, feel like, and be like a year from now. Then muse into what your life will look like two-years from now. Then imagine what you want your life to look like five-years from now. This is your future, success-story self. Allow all of your hopes and dreams into this vision of yourself, not just your health and weight loss goals.

Your future, success-story self is going to be by your side every day from now on. First you are going to create her. Then, you are going to have conversations in your head with her. This is actually really fun. Your future, success-story version of yourself will be with you throughout the day, thanking you, loving you up, and appreciating you for sticking with the SEXY diet every day. Your healthy, future self is going to be your biggest cheerleader and knows that you *can* and *will* succeed because your future self is already living the dream! Your future self is in awe of your strength. Create your success-story version of yourself right now. Once you have created your ideal version of yourself, you will be able to choose to operate from this personality whenever you want.

EXTERNAL HELPERS

You cannot do this alone. I encourage you to call upon a helper to be with you and guide you to stay on track so that you will achieve all of your health and weight loss goals. For many people, Jesus is their man.

Perhaps you would like to choose an angel, a spirit guide, the Universe, or a deceased relative. If you are uncomfortable with spirituality or religion, you may skip this step and invent another personality within yourself that will inspire you to stay on track to help you achieve ultimate success. For everyone else, it is deeply helpful to connect with your spiritual center and ask for guidance. Prayerfully declare your goals, hopes and dreams and ask that you be guided and held in love as you transform into the healthiest and happiest version of yourself. Asking for help from a spiritual source is a tool that will energize you and can offer grace when your willpower runs low.

HOW TO PUT THESE TOOLS INTO ACTION TODAY

When you have made a commitment to make big changes in your life, you want the changes to happen *now*. I know you are eager to get started and you want the weight to be off, like yesterday! The reality is that it takes time for the weight to come off. It takes a daily, and sometimes hourly commitment to your health. I want you to confidently know that you are sowing those seeds right now.

Your success in the SEXY Diet is largely going to be determined by your commitment to choose to be the healthiest version of yourself right now, in this red-hot moment. Take time, right now, to create your future, success-story self. First, imagine, in your mind's eye, what this new *you* looks like, then you visualize the heck out of it. Imagine it in your head or write it down in a journal. Imagine, in your wildest dreams, what your future self looks like. Create her and then invite this version of yourself into the driver's seat. Eventually you will morph into the image you have created.

Get specific! What does the scale say when you confidently step on it? How does it feel to pull on your favorite pair of jeans that fit perfectly and look great? How do you feel when you wake up every morning? What does it feel like to be hugged by your loved ones in this body? How does it feel to authentically smile when you look in the mirror? What does it feel like to really love yourself, inside and out? Where do you work? How do you spend your free-time? What new freedoms have you created in your life?

Create this new personality that you choose to become. Imagine into your future, success story-self, which is the version of *you* that has met all of your goals, hopes and dreams. Get very clear on what you look like and how you feel, because you are going to be talking to this version of yourself every day. Also, take time in prayerful meditation to ask for guidance in successfully achieving your ideal body weight and meeting all of your health goals from whichever spiritual source feels right to you.

I am so excited for you to have chosen to go on this transformational health journey. It is important for you to find pleasure in your weight loss efforts and the SEXY Diet will bring you tons of pleasure. Your first steps to transforming to your ideal body weight have already been taken. You are already on your way. Have fun with this!

CHAPTER 8

Self-Sabotage Masquerading as Self-Love

MY PERSONAL VERSION OF SEXY

The definition of Sexy, for me, is to be healthy and confident. I know I am healthy when I am following the SEXY diet and have tons of energy. Being confident means that I accept who I am unconditionally. Confidence means proudly celebrating all aspects of who you are: the good, the bad, and the ugly.

Luckily, we have a lot of confident role models in our culture. One for me is Amy Schumer. Amy Schumer is a famous American actress, comedian, and author. She is irreverent and can offend some people, but that girl can make me laugh! One of the things that I love most about Amy is that she truly accepts and loves her body, even though she does not have the body type that is typically celebrated in Hollywood.

I actually have no idea if Amy is healthy or whether she is at a healthy body weight. It is not my business nor is it my judgment call to make. It is Amy's business. I love that she is an empowered woman who has made the judgment call that she is worthy and awesome at her body weight, no matter what other people say. She has conviction and she can put the body-shamers in their place if they mess with her.

We were not all born with Amy's ability to find humor in every situation. Nor do we all have the conviction that we are worthy, no matter what others perceive our body weight to be. My wish for you is to cultivate the level of self-love and self-acceptance that Amy Schumer has. That said, there can be a shadow side to self-acceptance. What I am talking about is really not self-acceptance at all, rather, it is self-sabotage masquerading as self-love.

SELF-SABOTAGE OR SELF-LOVE?

When does self-love and acceptance turn into self-sabotage? It can happen very quickly and can easily be missed. I am going to tell you exactly how you can discern between the two so that you will avoid sabotaging your weight loss goals once and for all. Here is how you can identify when your level of self-love and self-acceptance has bled over into the territory of self-sabotage.

It is not always obvious at first, but you can always spot it when you realize that your ultimate goal, which is to transform into your future, success-story version of yourself, gets kicked to the curb, in the name of self-love. When you sabotage your goals in the name of self-love, it is not self-love at all, it is self-sabotage.

This has happened to me a million times, but there was this one time that I will never forget. It was the first time that I had made a commitment to go an entire week without eating sugar and flour. I was on day five, and I was feeling awesome. I was so proud of myself, and I remember thinking that I could go an entire month without sugar and flour. Then, I got a text message from a girlfriend, inviting me to a last-minute birthday party. I knew there were going to be a ton of temptations, but I held strong to my conviction that I would remain kibble-free at the party. But once I got to the party, all of my friends were drinking champagne and nibbling on these adorable mini cupcakes. The self-sabotaging voice in my head said, "it's OK to eat just one little cupcake. You have been *so* good these past five days. You've earned it!"

Has this every happened to you? Have you ever had a voice tell you to reward yourself with the very thing you know will make you feel bad? That, my friends, is self-sabotage masquerading as self-love. Yes, I *had* been a very good girl those past five days! But that does not give me the license to celebrate by sabotaging all of my goals! Self-sabotage is very sneaky and can happen quicker than you can open up your tool box, so you need to learn how to identify self-sabotage when it is happening, so you can quickly put her in the back-seat, and choose a better driver.

MULTIPLE PERSONALITY DISORDER

You have probably heard of Multiple Personality Disorder. They actually do not even call it that anymore, but most people have heard of Multiple Personality Disorder and have a wild image in their mind of what it looks like. I want you to take that image and imagine that we all have *multiple personalities*. Not a disorder, but rather lots of different personalities. I know this does not sound like the kind of tool you would want in your tool box, but trust me. This is a rad tool that you will use every day to lose all of your unwanted pounds!

The truth is, you do have multiple personalities. There are hundreds of personalities, identities and patterns of thought that you take on throughout any given day. Sometimes they come and go, and sometimes you choose which personality to bring forward. The tool itself is not *having* multiple personalities, rather the tool is knowing all of your unique personalities and *choosing* which one to intentionally bring forward. Choosing which personality to put in your driver's seat is a skill that you actually already have. I am just bringing your attention to it. This is an awesome tool in your tool box of success and I want you to get used to using this tool daily so that you can unleash the thinner, more empowered version of yourself daily. Choose to operate from the future success-story version of yourself that you created. When you choose to be the healthier version of yourself each and every day, you become that person. One day you don't have to choose it anymore, because it will become your primary mode of operation.

Some of your many personalities are self-sabotaging ones, while others are more aligned with self-love. I am going to detail a few of my sabotaging personalities so that you can better identify them in yourself and master the art of discerning between self-love and self-sabotage.

TYRANNICAL TODDLERS

Have you ever spent time with a toddler? I have had two of them, and they can be absolutely crazy. One moment they are sweet and kind and affectionate, and then, out of nowhere, they are screaming because they want the cracker *now*! Toddlers are crazy. But you know what, we were all toddlers once, and for some of us, this toddler behavior still lives somewhere deep inside of us. How many times have you had the overwhelming feeling that YOU NEED THE CRACKER NOW!!!

This is what I call my inner *Tyrannical Toddler*. You might have one too; I suspect most of us do. The inner *Tyrannical Toddler* puts you in a state of panic, where you cannot control your behaviors. You cannot reason with your inner *Tyrannical Toddler* because toddlers have no capacity for reasoning. Toddlers scream in the middle of grocery stores. They rage about crust on sandwiches and tiny brown spots on bananas. They are totally unreasonable. But we love them anyway. And they always eventually return to their sweet, lovable selves.

I suspect that for some of you, your emotional eating might be tied to your inner *Tyrannical Toddler*.

Any parent knows that yelling at her toddler when he is in one of his tyrannical frenzies only makes matters worse. We need to calmly and lovingly respond to our toddlers when they are in a tyrannical rampage. We also need to *not* give them the cracker NOW when they demand it, or we will create a monster. This has been a hard lesson for me to learn as a mom. But it is so important. When my toddler is tyrannically raging, I have to love him through his panic but not give in to his demands. I will hold him and happily cut the crust off when he has stopped screaming about it.

I have learned a lot about my own inner *Tyrannical Toddler* from my own children. When my inner *Tyrannical Toddler* rears her ugly head and starts demanding the chips and salsa NOW, I have learned to respond with love. I need to be loved even when one of my self-sabotaging personalities is in the driver's seat. That certainly does not mean I let my *Tyrannical Toddler* drive my car for long. I would have never let my 2-year old son drive my car in real life; and I am not going to let my inner *Tyrannical Toddler* run my life either.

But when my inner *Tyrannical Toddler* starts taking over, I know this is a sign that I need self-love. I need to accept myself. Your inner *tyrannical toddler* needs love too. She also need discipline. She needs to learn that it is not OK to scream every time she can't have a cracker.

It takes time for toddlers to get there, but most children stop throwing regular tantrums as they gain skills to manage their stress. We all have occasional set-backs. Adults sometimes throw tantrums too. The way to discipline an adult's inner *tyrannical toddler* comes from self-love and reaching for all of the tools in your tool box.

REBEL WITHOUT A CAUSE

I personally have a self-sabotaging personality that I call my inner *Teenage Rebel*. My inner *Teenage Rebel* frequently inspires me to sabotage my happiness. She is not all bad, in fact, sometimes she can be really fun, but she has definitely inspired some bad behaviors over the years. Obviously, she is younger than my biological age. She usually feels like a teenager, but sometimes she feels even younger. It is a little bit embarrassing to talk about her, but I am going to because I have gotten to know her pretty well over the years. My inner *Teenage Rebel* personality sneaks in from time to time and usually feels fun and free at first, but she is always getting me to do things I later regret. My *Teenage Rebel* said the word, "shit" on the playground when I was in elementary school. Now that I am a mom of two young boys, I do not think she is cool anymore!

My inner *Teenage Rebel* convinced me to drink alcohol at an age that was way too young and I spent two days barfing because of her. She said some embarrassing things when I was a Freshman in high school; she was trying to get me to impress an older soccer player. It was an epic fail, where I became the butt of my own joke, leaving this stud with the thought of me on the toilet. That was so not my intention! My inner *Teenage Rebel* feels kind of fun at first, but she has inspired me to do things that I have later regretted.

I remember feeling this inner *Teenage Rebel* personality a lot during my weight loss journey. She would always try to get me to drink too much wine when I was trying to avoid Miracle-Gro foods. She would try to reason with me, saying, "you have worked hard, now it's time to eat a huge basket of french fries because YOU DESERVE IT!"

Other times she would say, "why are you trying to lose the weight anyway? You should just love yourself just the way you are. Go and enjoy that second margarita and huge plate of nachos. You are way better than those idiots who judge others for being overweight!"

She would say, "You don't need to lose weight, you just need to love yourself as you are." She can sometimes be very sneaky. I can spot her though, because she is always trying to lure me away from my ultimate goal, which is to be my success story version of myself.

When an inner voice tells you that you should love and accept yourself just the way you are *and* to sabotage your health and weight goals in the same sentence, then that is a clear sign that the personality in the driver's seat is a self-sabotaging one, rather than a self-loving one.

Yes, we all could use more love and acceptance at our current body weight, no matter what that is. But loving oneself, does not mean giving up on making positive changes in your life. Accepting yourself as you are does not mean you are accepting that you are not going to get thinner or healthier.

This is a fine line to walk. It is easy to confuse self-love, self-care, and self-acceptance with self-sabotage. Yes, we need to love and accept ourselves now. At the same time, we also need to love ourselves enough to reach our health goals.

When your inner *Teenage Rebel* begins to tell you that you should just love yourself and not reach for your goals, remove her from the driver's seat. This is a tool that we already have in our toolbox: choosing which personality is making your life decisions. Make the choice to put your future, success-story version of yourself back in the driver's seat. Let your future, success-story version of yourself coach you through the difficult moments. Choose the healthier version of yourself right now.

YOU ARE A HOT MESS

Actually, you are probably not a hot mess, but sometimes I am. I have an inner *Hot Mess* personality that wears shorts that are way too short and has way too many "messy hair, don't care" days. I also have an inner *Sex Kitten*, but only my husband knows about her. I have an inner *Guru* who is totally in charge of writing half of this book. I have my inner *Quitter*, who is totally not allowed anywhere near the driver's seat while I am writing this book! I have an inner *Sociopath* who secretly fantasizes about castrating all of the convicted pedophiles that live within a one-mile radius of my home. I have an inner *Cinderella*, who is so terrified of being envied by other women, that I hide my successes and make myself unattractive anytime Cinderella gets near my car. I hate my inner Cinderella the most because she tortures me. When she's in the driver's seat, I fear that other women will hate me if they see my unique and beautiful qualities. When Cinderella is in the driver's seat, I try to make myself look unattractive and stupid so other women will not dislike me.

We all have tons of these inner archetypes and characters. It is so important that you start identifying your own inner characters and then dialogue with them. Get to know them. Ultimately, it is your choice whether to put them in the driver's seat. The better you get to know each of these gals, the good, the bad, and the ugly ones, the quicker you will be able to spot her when she's hijacked your car.

MY INNER CRAZY BITCH

Every once in a while, out of nowhere, my head explodes and F bombs fly out of my mouth like a drunken sailor. I rage on whoever the poor unsuspecting person is in my wake, probably my husband. In one minute, I am just your average super rad chick, and then suddenly I morph into a screaming lunatic. When my inner *Crazy Bitch* attacks my poor husband, you would have thought that he had just raped my dog and burned down our house because I am *that* mean to him. But in reality, the only thing he did was have the audacity to ask me if I know where his keys are.

I am sure this has never happened to you because you probably do not have an inner *Crazy Bitch*, like I do. But just in case you do, I want you to know that there is an antidote to this virus that seemingly attacks you from nowhere. The antidote? It's self-love. Are you starting to see a pattern? The antidote to your *Tyrannical Toddler*, your *Teenage Rebel*, your *Hot Mess*, your *Sociopath*, your *Cinderella,* your *Crazy Bitch*, and all of the others isn't to banish them. When we try to ignore them or suppress them, it only gives them more power. They are a part of us and we need to acknowledge them and give them some love. We do not want to give them power, just a little love.

When we temporarily transform into one of these familiar, ugly characters, they can easily derail us from our goals. My inner *Crazy Bitch* couldn't care less about achieving my ideal body weight. I cannot make good decisions when she is driving my car. But how do I get her out when she has hijacked my car for the fifth time this month? Acceptance and self-love. It sounds cheesy, but it's the freakin' truth!

You cannot banish you inner *Crazy Bitch* from planet earth. She's here. She is a part of you. The crazy thing is, she isn't trying to hurt you, she is actually trying to protect you. She is a wounded part of you and she needs love. She needs acceptance. She also needs to be told that she is not allowed to drive your car, because she's a terrible driver! You need to create healthy boundaries with these parts of you, in a loving way.

The reality is, you are not likely to reach for the tools in your tool box unless you have love and empathy for yourself. Self-love is a foundational tool and needs to be tended to, every day. If you do not know how to love yourself, start by loving a few little things about yourself. Start by celebrating a few of your favorite things about your life. Practice feeling grateful for just a couple of things about yourself that you are truly grateful for. Start by noticing a few things about yourself that you are authentically proud of. Plant these seeds of positivity and water them daily. A field of beautiful wild flowers will bloom and your self-love grow in this nourishing environment.

CHAPTER 9

The 6 Biggest Lies You Have Been Told

DEBUNKING WEIGHT LOSS MYTHS

You have been lied to. You have been told filthy, rotten, dirty, terrible lies your entire life, and these lies have broken your metabolism. It blows my mind how many weight loss myths are out there, masquerading as gospel. A quick google search on weight loss will result in an onslaught of metabolism slowing food choices and weight loss sabotaging techniques. Here are the six biggest lies that you have been told, your entire life, about how to lose weight. These lies need to be violently thrown in the garbage and smashed to pieces by an industrial size trash compactor. You are never, ever, going to make these mistakes again.

WEIGHT LOSS LIE #1: Breakfast is the Most Important Meal of the Day

Have you ever heard someone say, "breakfast is the most important meal of the day?" Of course, you have! That crap has been forced down your throat nearly every day since you were a child. The crazy thing is, there is not one clinical study to support it. There *is* a clinical study showing a correlation between people who eat breakfast and people who have better health markers and a slightly lower body weight. But *correlation* is very different than *causation*.

Eating breakfast does not magically make you healthy nor does it magically make you lose weight. The reason why breakfast is correlated with lower body weight is because the type of people who eat breakfast every day were also found to be more likely to avoid late night snacking. They were also more likely to exercise more. They had lots of other super healthy habits as well. There is much more to the story of eating breakfast than meets the eye. Breakfast is not any more important than lunch or dinner. What *is* important, is making better food choices.

WEIGHT LOSS LIE #2:
Eating 5-6 Small Meals a Day will Speed Up Your Metabolism

"Eating 5-6 small meals a day is good for your metabolism" is another weight loss lie that has been forced down our throats! Clinical Studies have put this one to rest: eating 5-6 meals a day does not result in a faster metabolism or more weight loss than eating 2-3 meals a day. In fact, eating more often can lead to more hunger.

So many so called, "experts" have said that it is somehow good for your metabolism to constantly feed it small meals throughout the day. But it is not. It is not *good* for your metabolism nor is it *bad*. The bottom line is that your metabolism does not need food every few hours to keep working. Just like your heart does not need food every few hours to keep beating. Your immune system does not need food every few hours to protect you from foreign invaders and your brain does not need food every few hours to keep processing information. Your body does not stop working when you stop eating food for a few hours, neither does your metabolism. Your metabolism actually speeds up when you give it periodic breaks from food, such as during intermittent fasting.

WEIGHT LOSS LIE #3:
Snacking is Healthy

Rarely do I see healthy snacking in my weight loss practice. Snacking is largely associated with poor food choices. Most conveniently packaged snacks, foods that I affectionately call, "kibble", are laced with the stuff we need to avoid for healthy weight loss: sugar, flour, and unhealthy vegetable oils. In addition to slowing down your metabolism, these foods damage your natural appetite-regulating systems. Also, snacking makes you constantly think about food. You ultimately want to gain freedom from obsessively thinking about food. Constantly snacking between meals does not set you free from emotional urges for food.

I am not saying that you cannot ever reach for a snack. There are days that I graze all day long! I just hope that if you do tend to frequently snack, you mindfully pack healthy snacks with you, such as cut up veggies, nuts, seeds, olives, or berries. If you want to graze through your day, stick to whole foods, not processed foods.

WEIGHT LOSS LIE #4:
You can eat Everything in Moderation

I hear people give this weight loss advice all the time. No, no and no! Throw this advice out the window! We don't smoke crack in moderation. Not everything is OK in moderation. The first problem with this weight loss lie is that moderation is highly subjective. My version of a moderate amount of dessert is likely very different than your idea of a moderate amount of dessert.

For weight loss, you do not need to eat perfectly all the time, but you do need to be more mindful of filling your belly with nutrient dense foods and cutting out the Miracle-Gro foods that slow down your metabolism.

This leads us to the second reason why this weight loss lie is so dangerous. A moderate amount of crackers every day will sabotage your entire weight-loss program. A cheat meal each week is expected. A cheat meal each day is not conducive to healthy weight loss. Stick to the SEXY diet most days and watch your metabolism speed up and your body fat melt away.

WEIGHT LOSS LIE #5:
Decrease calories and increase exercise to lose weight

This is my least favorite weight loss lie out there. You cannot exercise your way into your ideal pant size if you keep spraying Miracle-Gro on your fat cells. Sugar and flour put your body into a fat-storing mode and slow down your metabolism. You cannot exercise your way out of a bad diet. If you exercise a lot, while still eating the foods I offensively refer to as, "kibble", then your metabolism will slow down even more. You will have to increase your level of exercise just to maintain an overweight body.

I live in the Northern California Wine Country, which is a world-renowned cycling mecca. I see cyclists on the Wine Country roads all the time. I have no idea if they are locals or tourists, but I used to associate cycling with being really thin because cycling is known to burn a ton of calories. Plus, every competitor I have ever seen in the Tour de France has a body fat percentage that dreams were made of. But the reality is, most of the cyclist on the Wine Country roads do not look like the super lean guys riding in the Tour de France. I see big bellies and big booty's cycling around Wine Country every single day. I know that sentence just offended a ton of people, who will turn around and accuse me of "fat-shaming" the cyclists. My observation is not intended to fat-shame the cyclists. I am sincerely not making fun of these cyclist. I am simply stating an observation, which is that despite the fact that cyclists are burning a ton of calories on their rides, many still appear to live in a heavier body.

Another observation I have made is that I frequently see cyclist congregating at breweries in their cycling gear after their rides. What is it about cyclist and beer? I don't know, but it is totally a thing out here in Wine Country. Beer slows down your metabolism, as does pizza and granola bars, which are all things cyclist in Wine Country appear to love. The elite athletes competing in the Tour de France have sports nutritionists monitoring their diet, so they tend to eat less pizza and beer than the amateur cyclists. My point is, you cannot exercise your way out of a bad diet, no matter how much cycling or exercising you do.

WEIGHT LOSS LIE #6:
Fat Makes You Fat

Ok, I lied. *This* is my least favorite weight loss lie masquerading as truth. This one makes me so mad because fat can be so freakin' good for you! Healthy fats actually speed up your metabolism and stimulate the hormone that makes you feel full. Healthy fats help you avoid the real foods that make you fat, you know, kibble and the ones that spray Miracle-Gro on your fat cells.

Eating an excessive amount of calories can contribute to weight gain, but if you eat an excessive amount of calories in buttered broccoli versus an excessive amount of calories in crackers, the crackers are going to make you gain more weight, every time. Healthy fats include avocados, olives, nuts, seeds, extra virgin olive oil, coconut oil & grass-fed butter. Eat them in abundance!

Please spread the word so that no one else suffers sprains, bumps, breaks and bruises to their precious metabolism by following these outdated, harmful weight loss lies. Following the SEXY diet is your key to speeding up your metabolism and burning off all of your unwanted body fat.

CHAPTER 10

Burn Off the Calories You Overate Last Month, Today

Is it possible to burn off all of the calories that you overate last month, today? It is! I have one word for you: Fasting. Fasting is already in your tool box for successful weight loss. This chapter offers a thorough examination of all aspects of fasting and details exactly how to practice the art of intermittent fasting so that you will burn off all of your unwanted body fat.

FASTING VS. STARVATION

First and foremost, fasting is not starvation. I find it offensive when people equate fasting with starvation. Starvation is awful and happens in times of famine or war. We have all seen horrible images of children in war torn territories with distended bellies, hollow eyes and unimaginably tiny legs. Starvation has been used as a torture tactic throughout history and is a crime against humanity. Please, do not confuse fasting with starvation. Starvation is torture and leads to long-term metabolic problems and in many cases death. There is nothing funny about starvation, which is why I find it offensive when people joke about fasting as if it is "starvation". This minimizes the awful experience of those who have had starvation forced upon them. Fasting has nothing to do with starvation.

Fasting is defined as a period of time when an individual abstains from food. People abstain from food for spiritual reasons, health reasons, or to lose weight. While fasting, food is available; you are abstaining from food at your own will, and ideally you are eating a nutrient dense diet both before and after each period of fasting so that your body has all of the nutrients it needs for optimal performance.

Fasting is a choice; nobody is withholding food from you at any time. You are in control and you get to choose when to break your fast. Fasting can be very healthy and very safe. That said, it is important for everyone to be cleared by a health professional, such as your primary care physician, before starting fasting.

YOUR BACK-UP FUEL TANK

OK, I want you to grab ahold of your excess body weight right now. Just grab it! Grab your love handles, your thighs, your back fat, your belly fat or your arm fat. Squeeze it and feel it for a moment. Do you know what that is? That squishy fat in your hand is merely stored calories, waiting to be burned. Your body puts the excess calories you eat into your fat cells. It does this because it needs a handy place to keep the extra energy just in case you were ever to go a day or two without eating. Your body fat is nothing more than a back-up fuel tank.

Think of it this way: Your brain is always working, even when you are sleeping, so if you did not eat enough calories today, your brain is not going to stop working. It will just draw upon your stored fat cells to get the energy it needs. Typically, your body gets the fuel it needs from the food you eat today. But if you do not eat enough food today, your body will go to its backup fuel tank: your stored body fat.

What I am telling you is that you can either get your needed energy from the food you eat today or you can get your needed energy from your unwanted, excess body fat. Which would you prefer? I thought so!

When given the option, nearly everyone would *choose* to burn off their love handles and back fat to fuel their body's energy needs. The truth is, it *is* a choice and fasting is the tool you need to use when making that empowered choice. Fasting is the most efficient way to use your stored fat as calories. Again, you are not starving yourself. You have lots of calories stored in the fat all over your body. Your body can either get its needed calories from a meal right now, or from one you over-ate a few months ago. How rad is that?

DOES FASTING HURT YOUR METABOLISM?

Here is the biggest objection people make when it comes to fasting:

"But what about my metabolism? Won't my body go into *starvation mode* if I don't eat?"
There is that starvation word again. The answer is a firm "no". Your body does not go into *starvation mode* during a fast. In fact, your metabolism actually speeds

up when you fast! You read that right, fasting speeds up your metabolism!

The crazy thing is, restricting calories during a traditional diet makes your metabolism slow down. The only way to lose weight *and* speed up your metabolism is to fast. How excited are you to try fasting right now?

I do not recommend that anyone fasts for more than 24-hours. Doctors who specialize in medically supervised fasts tend to recommend that nobody ever fasts more than five days without medical supervision. That said, clinical studies have shown that your metabolism increases up to 14% during one to five day fasts. I am unaware of any clinical studies showing a slowing down of your metabolism from intermittent fasting. Fasting speeds up your metabolism!

HOW I LOST 30 POUNDS THROUGH INTERMITTENT FASTING

I am going to tell you exactly how I lost all of my excess body fat and how all of my private clients have successfully lost weight through intermittent fasting. I chose two non-consecutive days each week as my fasting days: I chose Mondays and Thursdays. I did not eat breakfast or lunch on Mondays and Thursdays. I did eat a healthy dinner on those two "fasting days". The other five days a week, I followed the SEXY diet. I enjoyed a cheat meal each week. And voila: the fat melted off of me and I have seen it happen again and again with all of my private clients.

Fasting is simple. Diets are hard because you have to restrict calories every single day. You are in a constant state of hunger, seven days a week. Cheat meals are rarely allowed because one cheat meal can blow an entire week of hard-core dieting. And then, after a couple of weeks of dieting, your metabolism slows down. How awful is dieting?

This is not the case with intermittent fasting. Fasting speeds up your metabolism and burns through your stored body fat.

WHO CAN FAST?

Nearly everyone can fast because we have been doing it for hundreds of thousands of years. Our bodies have evolved throughout thousands of years where humans have regularly experienced periods of feast and periods famine. We did not evolve eating three square meals a day. We have only been eating with this regularity for a little over a hundred years. How has that been working out for us? Do a quick google search on the obesity rate in America to get the answer to that question.

Intermittent Fasting is not a weight loss fad. Nearly every major religion advocates the spiritual benefits of fasting and our ancestors fasted regularly. Never in history have humans eaten three meals a day with snacks in between!

WHO CAN NOT FAST?

Pregnant women and children should never fast. Women who are breastfeeding an infant should not fast. People with Type 1 diabetes cannot fast. People with Type 2 diabetes can absolutely fast, as long as they do so under the supervision of their doctor and their blood sugar levels are monitored. People with a history of anorexia should not use fasting as a weight loss tool out of precaution so that one does not reactivate unhealthy behaviors.

That said, fasting has never been found to lead to disordered eating behaviors, such as anorexia or bulimia. Eating disorders have specific diagnostic criteria that have nothing to do with fasting. Anorexia has been classified by many experts as an anxiety disorder and has less to do with weight loss than managing issues related to control and anxiety. According to Dr. Jason Fung, an expert in intermittent fasting, fasting does not lead to eating disorders any more than washing one's hands leads to Obsessive Compulsive Disorder. You will not put yourself at risk for developing an eating disorder by practicing intermittent fasting. There are several clinical studies supporting evidence that intermittent fasting has never led to disordered eating. Disordered eating is beyond the scope of this book. If you suspect you have an eating disorder, please consider consulting your primary care physician and/or a psychologist.

Again, as with any change in diet or exercise, it is important to tell your primary care physician when you plan to make changes and try new things. Once you are cleared for fasting, you and your metabolism are going to love it!

It is really important to make healthier food choices whenever you are restricting calories for weight loss. Ideally, you are swapping out the foods I absurdly call, "kibble" and Miracle-Gro, with healthier choices on your non-fasting days, so your body is getting all of the vitamins, minerals, fats and proteins it needs to operate at its prime.

Just remember, your body is getting all of the calories it needs from your stored body fat. You will know, because your fat will begin to disappear immediately.

WHAT ABOUT HUNGER?

Hunger is not a sign that your body is in desperate need of calories or nutrients. You have all the calories you need in your stored body fat and if you are eating a nutrient dense diet, your body has built up enough of a supply of your micronutrients and macronutrients to get through your day. If you really think about it, you are only skipping four meals a week when practicing this form of intermittent fasting!

Hunger is often just a hormonal reaction that happens after eating certain foods. For instance, foods containing sugar and flour trigger your hunger hormone, ghrelin. Sugar and flour also make it harder to feel that feeling of being full after a meal. Hunger is not necessarily a signal that your body needs more calories, rather hunger can be a bad side effect from making poor food choices.

It is safe to feel hunger. If you are new to fasting, it might feel uncomfortable to feel hunger at first. We are not used to it, because we have been told to eat whenever we are hungry. We have been told to eat five to six small meals a day so it is likely that you are used to snacking regularly. Rarely do we feel hunger for longer than a few minutes because we are constantly feeding our hunger.

ARE YOU HUNGRY OR HANGRY?

The term, "hangry" means you are so hungry that you are angry. The feeling of being hangry is actually caused by large insulin dips after an insulin spike. What that means is that after eating bread, crackers, or sugar, your blood sugar goes up super high, and then crashes super low. The hunger you feel when the crash happens can actually make you angry. We rarely get HANGRY when we cut out sugar and processed foods and eat yummy veggies with healthy fat instead.

If you have not yet ditched the processed foods, it can make your fasting days harder. It is best to give yourself 24-48 hours of eating no sugar or processed foods before fasting, so your blood sugar is stable. It will make your fasting day a lot easier. Stay busy on your fasting days. I love fasting on busy working days, but if you do not work, schedule busy errand days and appointments on fasting days to make the time go by. Sitting in your home and staring at your refrigerator all day is not a good game plan. Each day that you successfully complete a fast, meaning you forego calories until dinnertime, you will gain more confidence in yourself and know that you can do it. Remember that fasting is safe and will speed up your metabolism at the same time as melting away your unwanted body fat.

I THINK I MIGHT BE HYPOGLYCEMIC

Fasting stabilizes blood sugar, so if you are someone who has *not* been clinically diagnosed with hypoglycemia, but find yourself using that word to describe yourself, you are probably scared of fasting because you feel changes in your blood sugar when you eat and when you don't eat.

Nothing changes your blood sugar more dramatically than sugar and processed carbs. You feel the dramatic changes in your blood sugar when you eat these foods. The law of gravity applies here: what goes up, must come down. When you eat food that dramatically increases your blood sugar, it comes down just as dramatically as it went up. What that means is that you probably feel really awesome right after you devour a cereal bar, but an hour later, you feel equally *not* awesome when the high has dropped. These highs and lows are not good for your body.

If you have not been clinically diagnosed with hypoglycemia, but you fear you need food every couple of hours because you feel your blood sugar drop, this blood sugar drop is likely caused by your food choices. Nothing will stabilize your blood sugar better than fasting.

What I am telling you is that unless your doctor has told you otherwise, fasting is right for you! Fasting stabilizes your blood sugar. It brings it down, and trains your body to keep it on the lower end, where you want it. Fasting will change your life and you will never want to throw around the word, "hypoglycemic" again!

IT IS SAFE TO SKIP A MEAL

It is absolutely safe to skip a meal and feel hunger. Here is a secret that most people do not know: The hunger you experience when you have not eaten in five hours and you are freakin' ready to devour your next meal, well, *this* hunger is actually more intense than the hunger you experience when you have not eaten in 72-hours. People anticipate getting hungrier and hungrier and hungrier to some sort of breaking point where their head explodes. Trust me, this does not happen. In fact, hunger waxes and wanes during fasting. It comes for a bit and then goes away, then it might return again. I always drink a tall glass of water when I experience hunger during a fast.

You know that feeling you get when you go to the gym and get a great workout in? I'm not talking about the post workout high, I'm actually talking about the pain you feel the next day, after you do 100 squats and your butt muscles are burning like crazy. If you are anything like me, every time you sit down and your glutes are on fire, you actually get excited because you know you had a great workout and you secretly feel like you gave yourself a Brazilian butt-lift.

Most people do not freak out that their muscles are sore after a workout because their sore muscles are actually feedback, telling them that they had an awesome workout. Hunger during a fast is the same thing. Your hunger is feedback from your body, telling you that you have burned through your available calories and that you are now burning fat as your calories. When you are fasting, you should be celebrating your hunger in the same way that you celebrate your sore muscles after a good workout.

FASTING FOR FAT LOSS

There are so many different ways to fast. There really is not one definition for fasting. In previous chapters, I detailed the fasting protocol where you eat only during a short window each day, such as six to eight hours every day. I find this to be a very effective strategy for weight maintenance and for balancing your circadian rhythms, but for profound fat loss, I encourage all healthy adults to try two, 24-day fasts on non-consecutive days each week, such as Mondays and Thursdays.

As soon as you have been cleared by your primary care physician to try intermittent fasting for fat loss, commit to two, non-consecutive days this week where you will skip both breakfast and lunch. The 24-hour fast actually begins the night before your fast, so you are sleeping during a good portion of your 24-hour fast. For example, if you choose to fast on Monday and Thursday of this week, then you would stop eating after dinner on Sunday night and break your fast at dinner on Monday night.

You are actually eating all seven days of the week. You are eating dinner all seven days. You are only skipping breakfast and lunch and snacks on Mondays and Thursdays. On your fasting days, you would eat a healthy 500-calorie dinner if you are a woman or a 600-calorie dinner if you are a man. You are totally allowed to drink coffee and tea on your fasting days, but definitely leave out the sugar. And drink lots of water.

I am not a doctor. You absolutely need to consult with a doctor, such as your primary care physician, before making any dietary changes, including integrating fasting into your life. I am really excited for you and your metabolism to try this life changing weight loss strategy known as fasting!

HEALTH BENEFITS OF FASTING

You are probably not going to fast because it is healthy for you, but just in case you wanted to hear about some of the health benefits that you are getting while you are burning off you unwanted body fat, I will list a few of them here.

Losing stubborn fat is my absolute favorite thing about intermittent fasting. My second favorite thing about intermittent fasting is autophagy. What? You've never heard of autophagy before? That's because nobody was talking about it until some dude won the Nobel Prize in Medicine for it in 2016. Autophagy is your body's self-eating system. The cells in your body actually eat the unhealthy part of itself when you are in autophagy. Autophagy is like spring cleaning for your cells. Autophagy occurs when the cells are starved of amino acids. It is actually their way of surviving when deprived of food. Instead of getting their essential amino acids, they eat the dysfunctional and dying parts of the cells when they aren't fed.

This is really interesting science. Cells are comprised of a variety of mini organs called organelles. Each cell has a nucleus, DNA, mitochondria, and protein areas. When you don't feed yourself food, your cells are denied the essential proteins they need to survive. Luckily, our bodies were magnificently designed in a way that expects we won't have access to food all the time. Never in the history of humans have we ever had access to food all the time, until the last 100 or so years. Our bodies have evolved to have this rad mechanism that makes your healthy cells literally eat the unhealthy cells when they don't have access to protein.

It turns out that fasting is the way your body does this naturally, which is why everyone should fast. Autophagy is your body's natural way of dusting away all of its unhealthy cells. Why would you want to do this? To slow down the aging process! Wrinkles are just aging cells showing their wear and tear. When you turn on autophagy, you dramatically slow down the aging process. Autophagy also encourages the growth of new, younger cells, so we look better and our brains work faster when we regularly initiate autophagy. Because the science of autophagy is relatively new, we are just learning about all of the benefits of autophagy, but studies are coming our regularly about the benefits of autophagy.

Autophagy is my favorite health benefit of intermittent fasting, but it isn't the only one. Fasting also speeds up your metabolism. It increases your growth hormone, which builds lean muscle. Fasting burns off belly fat and lowers blood pressure. The list of health benefits goes on and on. There are only side-benefits with fasting, no negative side-effects, unless you count hunger.

EXTRA SUPPORT

For some people fasting is very easy and natural, while for others it can feel very scary and hard. If you feel scared going into your first day of fasting, like I did, you need to find external accountability to get you through. You need to commit to another person that you are going to get through a day of fasting. The reason why having someone else hold you accountable is so effective is that it takes the heavy load off of you and gives some of the weight to the other person to carry with you. Fasting is much more manageable when you have another person there to help you carry the emotional load.

Fasting is both the most effective weight loss strategy of the SEXY diet, and is also the most challenging, especially when just getting started. Many people give up without proper support. I want you to succeed. I want you to be one of my success stories, so I offer courses that include an accountability group that will keep you on track. One of my programs includes a private Facebook community in addition to all the resources you need so that you will get all of the support you need to master the art of fasting. It takes the right mindset to get through a day of fasting. You need support. Join the community so that you can connect with other like-minded individuals who are also fasting for the first time.

Your future-self is so excited for you to begin this very safe and effective fat-loss tool known as intermittent fasting. It is absolutely the best thing I have ever done for my health and weight loss and I am so excited for you to get started.

Chapter 11

The Alien from Outer Space

THE "R" WORD

I was slower than the other children when I was
younger. I hadn't spoken a word by the age of two
and my mother was very concerned, so she took me
to the doctor. Up until now, I had assumed that my
mother had taken me to a pediatrician, but I am
beginning to wonder if she had actually taken me to a
proctologist, because this doctor was a total A-hole.
The doctor used a very offensive word when he
speculated possible diagnoses for a two-year old child
who hadn't yet spoken a word. He suggested I might
be, "retarded".

After hearing this very scary diagnosis, my
mother did what any other self-respecting hippie
would do in the late 1970's; she took me to a psychic.
The psychic my mother took me to was one of the
world's greatest psychics. I actually have no idea if she
had any gifts related to fortune telling, but she was
able to identify that my mother was extremely anxious
about this doctor's absurd diagnosis, and the psychic

took it upon herself to relieve this anxiety. This psychic went above and beyond the call of duty.

This psychic created an entire mythology around why I had not yet spoken while other children my age were stringing together three-word sentences. The day my anxious mother took me to the psychic, she learned that her precious daughter was slow, not because she was *retarded*, but because she was *special*. According to this brilliant psychic, I was sent to planet Earth from some distant planet to help all the Earthlings at this difficult time. The reason I could not speak, the mythology went, was because the language of this planet was unfamiliar to me and it would take me longer than the other children to pick up on the language because they had all reincarnated into this language many times before. The psychic then told my captivated mother all about the wonderful things I would do and all of the people I would help when I grew up.

My mother walked away with all of her anxiety relieved. The money used to hire the psychic was well spent and the psychic was vindicated when I finally began to speak, proving that horrible doctor wrong.

I DON'T BELONG HERE

I was fairly young when my mother told me this story. Actually, I was too young when my mother told me this story. My seven-year old brain was unable to discern between truth and mythology and I took the story very seriously. What my seven-year old mind heard, was that I was an alien from outer space.

I will never forget going to school in the first grade and telling my friend, April, that I am an alien from outer space. I was fully enrolled in my story. I completely believed that I was an alien from outer space, so I was surprised to see her stunned reaction. I quickly told her not to worry, I was a good alien and that I came here to help people, but the last thing I remember is watching April skipping away, off to go play with another child. April and I did not remain friends throughout elementary school.

There was a point in high school where the memory of being an alien from outer space crept up on me and I put the pieces together. I realized that the psychic had made up this entire narrative about me to ease my mother's anxiety, rather than having psychically received this interplanetary information. I was kind of pissed at my mom for being so gullible as to believing the psychic. But mostly I was ashamed for having been so gullible myself for believing that I was special.

I believe that the psychic's intentions were good, but harm had been done. I had developed an inner story about myself that constantly reinforced a belief that I do not belong here. I believed deep down, at a subconscious level, that I am not an Earthling. I have always felt that I am different than everyone else.

When I had a difficult time with a subject in school, I felt like the other kids had it easier because they were learning something that they had already learned, in a past life, whereas I was having to learn everything for the first time. But mostly, I felt like I did not belong here and that I am only here, on planet earth, in service of others. I was confused about what my mission was, but I knew there was a mission.

Never did I feel like a member of planet earth. I have always carried a feeling that I am just a visitor in a strange land. I grew up feeling that I do not belong in any group. This was validated by the fact that I never fit in with any clique at school. I was always able to make friends, but I did not have my own inner circle.

WE BELONG TOGETHER

The truth is, we all belong. This mythology of separation is everywhere. Sadly, I am no more special than others in holding this deeply seeded belief that I do not belong. Immigrants have written scores of books on the feeling of not belonging. Children of adoption, minority communities, LGBTQ, inter-religious couples, people with disabilities, and just about everyone who has ever experienced the perception of feeling different than the majority have a story in their head that they do not belong.

The reason why I am bringing this up in the middle of a book about weight loss is that I hear over and over again in my practice that women who consider themselves overweight, feel like they do not belong. I know that my excess weight intensified my feelings of not belonging.

Girlfriend, you *do* belong and never let anyone tell you otherwise. You belong here on planet earth. You belong to your family. You belong to your country, your community, your church, your husband's family, your yoga class, even if you are the least flexible yogi in the class and you belong in your art class, even if you are the worst artist in the class. You belong, regardless of whether you are the best or the worst. You belong, even though you are different. And yes, you are very different than those around you. You are undoubtedly very different than everyone else around you, but you still belong. You are still a valuable member of this group and you are every bit as important as everyone else.

I have now made peace with being an alien from outer space. I sometimes fantasize that this psychic did have access to some interplanetary information and that I *am* a newbie at this Earthling thing, here in service of helping others. I have come to like this magical story. I hope I carry out this special mission and am granted the opportunity to stay a few lifetimes here on this gorgeous planet with all of these rad Earthlings that I have had the pleasure of meeting.

What I have learned on this planet is that we are all special. We are all beautiful souls of great importance and we all have the opportunity to contribute to the betterment of this magnificent, blue planet that we have the luxury of calling home. We all belong here and we all matter, no matter what.

CHAPTER 12

How to Speed Up Your Metabolism

I HAVE NEVER EXERCISED AS MUCH IN MY LIFE AS I DID WHEN I WAS AT MY HEAVIEST

Let me share a very personal story. I was getting married in September of 2009 and I was not even close to my ideal body weight in 2009. My elliptical machine & Pilates classes alone were not cutting it and I was so frustrated. The local YMCA is only 3 blocks from my house and they were running a summer special. I signed up so I could add spin classes to my exercise regime and lose weight for my wedding day.

I vividly remember my spin class at the YMCA. It was awesome. The spin room smelled kind of bad, but besides that, I loved it. I would always leave with shaking legs and soaking wet from sweating so hard. I was burning tons of calories in that class! But what really struck me was the instructor. She was a great motivator and played really fun music, but what really stood out for me is that she lived in a heavier body. I did not know her story, other than she taught several spin classes each week, so I assumed that she and I would both be losing weight during that summer leading up to my wedding.

I exercised like crazy that summer. I went to spin class twice a week, I paid a fortune for private Pilates classes twice a week, I worked out three days a week on my elliptical machine and I walked my dog at least twice a day. That is truly a lot of exercise! I went to my last spin class three days before my wedding day. To my disappointment and surprise, neither the spin instructor nor I appeared to have lost a significant amount of weight all summer long.

How was it that we were both exercising like crazy, but not dropping any weight? Why was it so damn hard to lose weight?

I never went to spin class again after my wedding day. My elliptical machine began collecting dust because I gave up. It is so frustrating to exercise like crazy and count your calories and not lose weight. Weight loss plateaus SUCK. What I did not understand then is that cutting calories and exercising usually results in a slower metabolism.

HOW TO SPEED UP YOUR METABOLISM

What is your metabolism anyway? It is not a body part, like a pancreas or a liver, rather it is a process. It is the process of turning calories into energy to fuel your body. Your basal metabolic rate is usually what people mean when they refer to their metabolism. This is the number of calories your body uses just to keep you alive. You need a certain number of calories to keep your heart beating, lungs breathing and your brain cells firing. Without any effort on your part, your body will naturally burn your basal metabolic rate of calories just to keep you alive. In case you were wondering, clinical studies have shown that your basal metabolic rate does not decrease when you practice intermittent fasting.

Your metabolism also allocates calories to digest the food you eat and it allocates calories for movement, whether exercising at the gym or chasing your toddler around or sauntering to your car from the grocery store. Every day you use a certain number of calories to move around.

If you are consuming the number of calories required by your body to maintain your body weight, let's pretend that number is 2,000 calories for easy math, the breakdown is as follows: Your basal metabolic rate takes an astonishing 60-75% of the calories you burn every day. That's 1,200-1,500 calories just to keep your lungs breathing, heart beating, immune system functioning and brain cells firing. You burn approximately 10% of your calories just to digest your food, so that's about 200 calories a day. The remaining 15-30%, which is 300-600 of your daily calories are used performing your daily activities, like walking.

HOW NOT TO SPEED UP YOUR METABOLISM

The most efficient way to lose weight is *not* through exercise. In order to burn 600 calories, you need to jog for a good two hours. The best way to flood your body with the dread hunger hormone is by jogging for two hours. Nearly everyone who exercises at that level compensates by eating more.

Everyone's metabolism is different. The average person expends anywhere between 60-75%

of their daily intake of calories on their basal metabolic rate, that is if you are eating the number of calories *your* body needs to maintain your weight, not gain or lose weight.

So, here is the Million Dollar question: "Is there a way to change your basal metabolic rate?" The answer is a complicated yes. The answer lies in your hormones, which are affected by your food choices.

THE BIGGEST LOSER

Are you familiar with the TV show The Biggest Loser? It is a reality competition where individuals compete to lose the most weight. I have always found the title of this TV show to be offensive because the title appears to be a double entendre, suggesting that overweight people are losers. Now that I have the knowledge of the harm they are doing to the poor contestants, I am even more disgusted by this TV show.

The brilliant Dr. Jason Fung points out that what sets the Biggest Loser apart from all other reality shows is that they never have a reunion show. They never have a reunion show because something like 95% of the contestants have regained a significant amount of weight back; many contestants weigh more now than when they started the show. Why is that? Why do all of the contestants on the Biggest Loser eventually gain a significant amount of weight back after working so incredibly hard to lose it? It is not because they are bad people. It is not because they get lazy or return to eating massive quantities of junk food after the show ends. It is because the way they are told to lose weight on the show slows down their metabolism.

When you continue to eat food that is like Miracle-Gro for your fat cells, such as convenient, "low-calorie" foods like protein bars, cereal bars, health bars, you know, *kibble bars*, you slow down your metabolism. Remember, these convenient, processed foods that I absurdly refer to as kibble, instantly usher your calories into your fat cells. This Miracle-Gro effect prevents you from burning fat as energy; you instantly go into fat-storing mode when you are spraying your fat cells with their version of Miracle-Gro: sugar and flour. To add insult to injury, these foods flood your body with the dreaded hunger hormone, so you walk around in a constant state of hunger.

Even if the food is labeled *whole wheat flour* or *corn flour*, it is a refined food. You want to avoid anything labeled *flour*. The reason flour is bad for you is because they remove the naturally occurring protein and fat from the wheat or the corn or whatever grain they are turning into flour. Then they grind it up into an extremely fine powder, and the resulting product mimics that of sugar when it hits your blood stream. Flour is basically sugar as far as your body is concerned. This is why the S in SEXY includes flour along with sugar. They are both powerful fertilizers for your fat cells.

HOW EXERCISE CAN SLOW DOWN YOUR METABOLISM

Yes, exercise can actually slow down your metabolism. Crazy, right? Everyone has told us that exercise speeds up your metabolism. And it can. But it doesn't always. It depends on what foods you are eating. Sugar and flour are once again the culprits. These foods act like a prison-guard who forces all of your calories into your fat cells and then locks them in forever, throwing away the key. If you are eating sugar and processed carbs every day, like bread or soda, you become a perpetual fat-storing machine.

Exercise cannot put you back into a fat-burning mode because these foods override exercise. I used to hear all the time that exercise speeds up your metabolism. But the reality is, exercise can actually slow down your metabolism, if you are eating processed foods. This revelation blew my mind. Is your mind blown? I am still furious that I exercised as much as I did, and all I was doing was slowing down my metabolism! I thought I was speeding it up, but the scale does not lie.

If you are exercising like crazy, like they do on the Biggest Loser, your body needs calories to fuel your brain, your immune system and all of your systems. Your body is searching for calories but it cannot find any calories because insulin is a greedy bastard who will not share any of his calories with the rest of your body. He's holding all of your calories prisoner, inside your fat cells. Your body eventually goes into emergency shut-off mode, meaning it slows down your metabolism to compensate for the lack of available calories. This is why all conventional diets result in the dreaded weight loss plateau followed by gaining all of the weight back.

95% OF ALL DIETS FAIL

The numbers are astonishing. It is estimated that between 95-98% of all diets fail. They all lead to the dreaded weight-loss plateau, followed by gaining all of the weight back. Initially, your body will release weight when you restrict calories or increase your exercise. But after a short period of time, the insulin (a-hem Miracle-Gro) will lock it in. If you are eating sugar and flour, your body will not be able to shed any more pounds, putting you into a weight loss plateau. Even though you cut more calories or burn more calories through exercise.

Then, your poor brain and immune system and all other systems are like, "Hey there! We need some more calories to keep working!"

And your body is like, "Um, I can't find any." Even though you have just eaten a ton of calories. Those calories are being held prisoner, locked inside your fat cells. Instead of shutting your brain down, your body just allocates less calories to your brain and everywhere else. The crappy cherry on top is that you are then flooded with the dreaded hunger hormone, in a desperate attempt to get more calories. This is the slowing down of your metabolism. Your brain is now forced to function on less calories than is ideal, your metabolism has literally just slowed down, and, to make matter worse, you are feeling ravenously hungry all the time because your body is drowning you in hunger hormones. It is truly a vicious cycle.

HOW LAUREN LOST 60 POUNDS

My client, Lauren was experiencing exactly this when we started working together. She weighed 183 pounds when we first met and had been at a weight loss plateau for months, despite the fact that she was restricting calories to only 1,200 a day while exercising with a personal trainer 3 times a week and diligently doing her cardio. She was really strong from her workouts, great muscle tone, underneath a significant amount of excess body fat.

She was doing everything that conventional wisdom had informed her to do: She was eating less calories and moving more. She was stuck in a frustrating weight loss plateau and she was about to go into another predictable weight gain cycle, but luckily she started working the 4-part proven weight loss system known as the SEXY Diet.

First, I removed the flour and sugar from her diet and increased her daily caloric intake by including healthy fats and nutrient dense foods. I also had her fast two non-consecutive days each week.

HER WEIGHT LOSS PLATEAU VANISHED IMMEDIATELY

Within 8 months, Lauren had lost 60 pounds and now knows how to maintain a healthy body weight. Lauren did not think it was possible to get to 123 pounds. She was hoping to get to around 150 pounds. But once she got there, she realized how easy it was to shed the pounds by working the SEXY diet. She was not satisfied with the amount of body fat she still had around her midsection, so she stuck with the program.

My proudest moment working with Lauren was not the day the scale hit 123 pounds. My proudest moment was when she messaged me and said, "Summer, I have never felt so much energy in my life. I feel amazing. I feel like I can fly. I feel like I can do anything!" By shedding the unwanted weight and speedup up her metabolism, she regained her youthful energy. She chases her toddler around with profound energy. She loves the way she looks, but she really loves the way she feels.

The good news is that you can immediately speed up your metabolism by shifting your hormones. You do this by avoiding foods like sugar and flour, that spike your body's Miracle-Gro. You can simply replace one processed carb or sugar-fest meal today with a healthier alternative. Your metabolism will immediately love it and reward you by working faster. Eat the rainbow. Choose lots of vegetables and dress them with healthy fats such as extra virgin olive oil and coconut oil. If you want to supercharge it, then throw in a couple of fasting days. Fasting completely eliminates this Miracle-Gro like hormone from your body. When you fast, instead of getting today's caloric needs from today's meals, you are getting them from a meal you overate a few months ago. How cool is that?

CHAPTER 13

Synchronicity

How did you find this book? I imagine, like most, you have a story about what led you to discovering this book. Your story undoubtedly has elements of synchronicity in it. The word synchronicity means, "meaningful coincidences". For many, a synchronicity is seen as an affirmation that external forces are working in their favor. For others, a synchronicity validates that they are on the right path, like a wink or thumbs-up from God. Synchronicity is a sequence of favorable events that occur when we are "in flow", following our hearts and intuition.

I learned about synchronicity from my mother, Peyton. Peyton always seemed to find herself smack dab in the middle of these amazing synchronicities!

My mother was diagnosed with breast cancer when I was only 11 years old. She beat it, but when I was 14 years old, she began having tremendous pain throughout her body. After getting a CT scan, a doctor told her that he had both bad news for her and good news. The bad news was that her breast cancer had metastasized to her bones. The good news was that she had one year to live. Clearly, he was a jerk.

My mother had Christian Scientist influences growing up, and while no longer practicing, she held strong beliefs in the power of positive thought for healing. She never believed that she would live only one more year, despite what the doctor had told her. She vowed to live long enough to see me graduate from high school. She turned her attention toward meditation, prayer, and positive thinking. She accepted some of the Western medicines offered to her, but rejected others that her intuition told her to avoid. She profoundly believed in her body's ability to heal.

I am grateful to report that my mother far exceeded her goal to live to see me graduate from high school. Not only did she beat the cancer a second time, but she lived cancer-free for over ten years before the cancer returned a third time.

SYNCHRONICITY

About a year before her death, my mom was fortunate to be put into a "study" at UCSF Medical Center at Mount Zion. The tumors were not responding to the FDA approved medicines that were on the market at the time, so her oncologist referred her to a study using experimental medicines in San Francisco with the hopes of slowing the tumors. Fortunately, this experimental medication worked and bought her a precious extra year with us.

The oncologists in San Francisco administered the experimental medication on a very rigid schedule. They would give her an infusion of the medicine every Tuesday, for three straight weeks; the fourth Tuesday of the month, she was given off to rest. Then the next month would begin and she was back in the infusion room, every Tuesday, for three consecutive weeks. We did not live in San Francisco, so three Tuesday's a month, my mom, my grandpa and I would all drive to San Francisco, cross the Golden Gate Bridge, turn up Divisadero Street until we reached UCSF, and then take the elevator up to the 5th floor to the infusion room where my mother would receive the cutting-edge cancer treatment.

The infusion room in San Francisco was much bigger than the one in our hometown. There were a lot more patients and nurses and they provided a wider variety of refreshments in the waiting room. The walls were covered with beautiful art and they even had guitarists gently play music for the patients. It was a much different experience than going to the infusion room back in our hometown.

During the time that my mother was receiving these cancer treatments, she and her husband, Mikey wanted to go to the annual Mendocino music festival. My mom was elated when she discovered that the week of the music festival corresponded with her week off from her treatment at UCSF! They immediately booked their favorite rental home in Mendocino overlooking the ocean and bought four tickets to the night of the music festival that a specific performer that she loved was playing; their best friends were going to join them for a few days and they all planned to go to the music festival together.

Unfortunately, their friends had to cancel last minute, leaving my mother with two extra tickets to this show. The music festival had been sold out for several weeks, so my mother was not worried about finding someone to give the tickets to. She just wanted to find the *right* person to give the tickets to. My mother was a very giving person and the idea of selling the tickets never crossed her mind, she wanted to gift them to a deserving person; she patiently waited for the *right* person to come along. Each day of their vacation went by, and each day she did not find anyone to give these two coveted tickets to. She was not worried though; she knew in her heart that she would eventually find the *right* person.

The Friday evening of the concert came. My mom and Mikey had reservations at a restaurant for dinner that happened to be a block away from the huge white tent where the concert was taking place. She arrived at the restaurant with all four tickets, still convinced that she would find the *right* person to give the tickets to, and found that the restaurant had pushed the tables closer together than usual in order to accommodate more tables.

It was a very busy night in the town of Mendocino, filled with excited concert goers. Shortly after they were seated, another couple was seated at a table right next to theirs. Because the tables were so close together, it was easy for my mom to strike up a conversation with this couple.

"Oh, you must be going to the show tonight!" My mom said.

"I wish we could go, we tried to get tickets, but the show was sold out!", responded the man.

"Wow, that's too bad, it's going to be an amazing show!", said my mom.

"I know! I'm a musician and I have always wanted to see this band!"
My mother's heart began to tingle, she was sensing that she finally found the *right* people to give the tickets to, when the man said, "We just drove into

Mendocino today from San Francisco. We just got married! We are now officially on our honeymoon!"

With tears in her eyes and a tingling sensation all over her body, my mom joyfully said, "Well, today is your lucky day. I happen to have two extra tickets and would love to give them to you for your wedding present."

The newlyweds were astonished and incredibly grateful. After they finished their dinners, the four of them walked to the show together.

At intermission, my mother felt that there was something unfinished; she had a feeling that there was some sort of connection she had with the man, and felt compelled to learn more about him. She asked him to tell her more about himself. He told her,

"I've been a musician in San Francisco all of my life; I play guitar, compose music and teach guitar lessons, but my passion is in the community service that I do. Every Tuesday, I play guitar for the cancer patients on the 5th floor at UCSF."

As I write these words, with tears in my eyes, I can only imagine how my mother felt in that moment. She told me that she froze and was rendered speechless. After a few moments, she was able to compose herself and found the words to tell this incredible gentleman that she was one of the cancer patients that had been blessed by his music every Tuesday at UCSF. Together, they marveled at this synchronicity.

After that night, my mother never saw this man again. The experimental drug stopped working for her and she was taken off of the study, but she was profoundly grateful that she was able to give something back to a great man who had selflessly offered her comfort so many times before.

Some people will say that this was all just a coincidence. Honestly, I feel sorry for people like that. God moved mountains to bring my mother and this man together at this exact beautiful moment in the small coastal town of Mendocino. It is unfortunate to live a life where you cannot see the miracles that are literally taking place right in front of you.

You can tell the difference between a synchronicity and a coincidence because synchronicities are much more powerful and emotionally impactful. They bring deeper meaning and richness into our lives and remind us of our blessings. Synchronicities are validations from beyond and affirm that we are on the right path.

You *are* on the right path. Synchronicities are all around you. I believe you are in the middle of a great synchronicity right now and something magical is right around the corner. I have a deep sense that my mother now dances among the angels of synchronicity. When you need grace in your life, when you need a magical intervention, say a prayer to Peyton and the angelic ones who orchestrate synchronicity. You will be amazed to see the mountains that move in your favor. I encourage you to breathe in the remarkable synchronicities in your life. May the synchronicities continue to validate and guide you on your great path.

CHAPTER 14

Become an Alchemist

THOUGHTS ARE THINGS

Dr. Bruce Lipton, the brilliant stem-cell biologist, teaches that thoughts are things. He eloquently lectures about how thoughts are actually frequencies. Your thoughts communicate with the receptors in your cells; these are the exact same receptors that your hormones communicate with. Your thoughts actually tell the receptors on the cell membrane what DNA to make. Your DNA then communicates with your RNA, and that communication results in the decision of what proteins you make. Stay with me here, because you are going to want to hear this. These proteins actually decide what makes *you*. You are literally made of the proteins that your thoughts have initiated making. Your thoughts literally decide whether you make dopamine or serotonin, or a fast metabolism or a slow one.

YOUR THOUGHTS BECOME YOUR DESTINY

Your biology and ultimately your destiny are made by the thoughts you are thinking. The fact is that your biology comes from your beliefs and your thoughts. Energy is communicated from your thoughts to your cells. This is proven by science! Thoughts transform your cells. You become your thoughts! What thoughts are you telling your body to make every day? Are you telling your body that you have a slow metabolism or are you telling your body that you are a fat burning, sexy beast?

Your mind and your body are linked. You cannot separate them, nor can you change one without changing the other. Your thoughts, whether positive or negative, literally enter your DNA, epigenetically. Over time, with our thoughts, we have the ability to become a new person. Along with a healthy diet, we can fast track this!

This is why thoughts of greatness and success are so powerful. If you plant a watermelon seed, you will get a watermelon, every time. You will never get a tomato from a watermelon seed. The same principle applies to your thoughts. If you plant positive seeds in your mind, positivity will grow in your life. You have the power to control your thoughts, which is why you are the master of your fate. Your dominant thoughts become your reality. Download positive programming into your subconscious any way you can, as often as you can! Remind yourself daily that you are worthy, you are loved, and that you are a soul of great importance in the universe. You will change your DNA and ultimately who you are. Practice positive thinking so that you can create the body and health of your wildest dreams!

ENERGY CANNOT BE CREATED NOR DESTROYED

But what about those negative thoughts? Are they really harming you? The truth is that negative energy is not solely bad. It is powerful and can be transformed into positivity. The practice of transforming negative energy into positive energy is modern day alchemy. Instead of turning lead into gold, we are transmuting negative energy into positive energy because negative emotions have great energy. Do not waste this energy, rather use it! All emotions hold power that you can use to your benefit. Apply it in a positive way; transform the energy! Emotions can transmute into useful capacities, which is one path of discovering treasure underneath your pain.

For instance, sadness and grief can be transmuted into compassion. Anger can be transformed into fierceness. Shame can be transformed into dignity and humility.

It is important that you transmute these challenging emotions so that you cultivate more positivity while creating a life of ease and flow. How do you go about the work of transmutation? There are three key elements to transmuting your negative emotions into positive capacities.

ALCHEMY: TURN YOUR LEAD INTO GOLD

STEP 1: Cultivate Awareness

The first step of transmuting your negative emotions into powerful capacities is self-awareness. The opposite of self-awareness is blaming everything that happens to you on everything else. We all know people like this, they have absolutely no sense of personal responsibility and blame everyone else for their problems. I knew another mom from my son's preschool who would constantly whine about her boss, her husband, her neighbor, her mother-in-law and even her Congressman. People who blame everyone else for their problems are obnoxious to be around. We all know a person like this. They have no insight that they are actually responsible for a lot of their happiness. They go through their disempowered life, constantly blaming everybody else for every little thing that goes wrong. This person lacks self-awareness. Don't be like her.

Self-awareness is not only about taking personal responsibility. You must also be aware of your negative self-talk and negative belief systems. You do this by stepping outside of yourself when you are feeling an emotional trigger, and observe your thoughts and feelings. Instead of reacting from a place of negative feelings, stop, breathe and observe these thoughts and feelings so that you can respond from a higher place, like your inner *guru*, instead of your inner *tyrannical toddler*.

It is also helpful to journal about your negative self-talk and negative feelings. Dig deep and discover how long you have been carrying around your negative patterns. It will be tremendously helpful to identify where the negative beliefs associated with the negative emotions stem from. Did you pick these beliefs up from your parents, peers, spiritual leaders or teachers? Many of your negative beliefs are commonly held in our culture; when we transmute these negative cultural beliefs within ourselves, we can free others from the shackles that bind them.

STEP 2: Cultivate Empathy

Empathy is the capacity to feel into another person's awareness. The art of cultivating empathy begins with allowing yourself to be affected by what others are going through. You need to feel your own emotions as well as feel into what another might be going through. You cannot develop an empathic stance if you stand back, aloof and unaffected by other people's experiences. In order to develop your empathic muscle, you must take yourself out of your own shoes and imagine putting someone else's shoes on.

It's kind of like putting on your husband's stinky shoes for a minute to find out why he's in such a foul mood. You do this by taking off your cute wedges, then slip into his disgusting shoes, and imaginatively walk a mile in them. When you do this, you realize his life kind of sucks today, so that's why he is in such a pissy mood. Stepping out of your perfectly fit shoes and into his awkward, bulky shoes, reminds you that, wow, he *did* have to get up at 5am today to give a presentation at work, and then got yelled at by his boss when the PowerPoint presentation failed, only to come home to a wife who is annoyed that he forgot to take out the trash again. Suddenly, you realize that you would much rather take

out the trash in your cute wedges than have to deal
with the stress he's dealing with in his stinky shoes.

Wouldn't it be nice if your partner took off
his shoes every once in a while and walked a mile in
your wedges? I can't help you in that department, but
I have another solution for you. What if *you* tried it?
What I mean is, what if you pretended that you
weren't really you for a moment, but an outsider
looking in at your life. What would they think of you?
My guess is that they would have a lot of compassion
for what you have gone through in your life. Can you
find a way to have that level of compassion for
yourself?

It is just as important to have empathy for
yourself as for others. Sometimes you need to look at
yourself from the outside and cultivate a little more
empathy for all that you do. It can be much easier to
feel empathy for others than for yourself. Little by
little, you can develop more empathy for yourself by
imagining you are someone else, looking into your
life. Another way to look at it: would you love and
care about another person if they were in your shoes?

STEP 3: Seek Accountability

Have you ever tried to carry a couch up a flight of
stairs all by yourself? That is a silly question. It would
be nearly impossible to carry a bulky, heavy,
rectangular object up a flight of stairs all by yourself.
You need a strong partner to stand at the other end
of the couch to carry half of the burden. You need a
competent partner to help navigate the difficulty of
getting the heavy piece of furniture up the stairs,
illuminating your blind spots when you cannot see the
next step in front of you. When you have a partner,

together, step by step, you can carry the couch up the stairs until you reach the top. This is exactly how external accountability works. When you have a monumental goal to meet, the finish line looks impossible when you are standing at the bottom of the stairs, all alone. You often don't even know how to get physically started, not to mention the heavy emotional load that is bogging you down. It can be nearly impossible to reach your goals when you are all alone. An external accountability partner takes on half of your burden, and makes it manageable. They walk with you up the stairs, step by step, carrying half of your emotional load, championing you along the way. Your accountability source reminds you of your strength, illuminates your blind spots and keeps you focused on each step, until you reach the top.

Everyone needs accountability to stay on track so that they meet their goals. This can look like sharing your experience with a friend, but more frequently this looks like seeking external counsel. The need to share your experience in community is part of your human nature. External accountability works because sharing your experience with another opens you up to being seen as your future success-story version of yourself. Your accountability person knows that you can do it. An external accountability source reminds you of your goals when you forget, keeps you on track, day in and day out and believes in you when you stop believing in yourself. Your success rate skyrockets when you have an external accountability source.

INFORMATION VERSUS TRANSFORMATION

In this book, I am giving you everything you need to know to speed up your metabolism and burn off all of your unwanted body fat. I am literally giving you all of the information that you need. I am not withholding any information with the intention of giving you the final information that you need in one of my paid programs. I can do this, without putting myself out of business, because there is a profound difference between information and transformation.

This is an important distinction, so please do not skip over this part, because I want to ensure your success on your weight loss journey.

You do not need more information, rather you need a transformation. We live in the information age and get all the information we need for free on the internet. I personally give nearly all of my teachings away for free in my vlogs, book and TV show. It is empowering to have the information you need to make change. But information rarely leads to change. Let me repeat that so that it will sink in. Information does not lead to change. What you need is *transformation*.

TRANSFORMATION FOR THE WIN

This begs the question, "what transforms when we are transforming?" In my online program, I am not only transforming your metabolism and body weight, but I am also looking to transform your consciousness. Without a transformation of your consciousness, you will not change old habits. You may try out a few things that you have learned, but it will not lead to life-long changes, until you have a transformative experience.

This is why I include countless techniques and practices within the chapters of this book. They contain the experiential component that you need to succeed. The tools and practices that I include are all designed to transform your consciousness, so that you will never slip back into old patterns and habits that have harmed you and kept you unhealthy and overweight. I give you practices so that you will gain the benefit of a whole body and soul transformation.

You must do the practices in the book in order to transform your consciousness, your body and your metabolism. Some readers will engage with the practices and techniques outlined in the book, while others perform better with external accountability, and will need to join one of my programs in order to ensure that they will have a life-changing transformation. You can make that decision for yourself by monitoring your results. If the transformation is going slower than you would like, then you are a strong candidate for a program that will give you the accountability you need to transform into your future, success story version of yourself.

HOW TO HAVE AN EPIC TRANSFORMATION

Your success is largely going to be determined by your commitment to choose to be the healthier version of yourself right now. I know that is a lot of words. It means that you will be successful if you choose to make the healthier choice in every moment.

Well, how do you do that? How do you choose to be the healthier version of yourself every day? How do you ensure that you will be one of the people reading this book that will transform into your future, success-story version of yourself?

It is not just about eating healthy and fasting, because if it really was that easy, everyone would be at their ideal body weight. Most people begin strong. They will initially eat healthy and fast, but then something will happen and they slowly stop eating healthy and stop fasting. Why is that? Why do most people get derailed from their goals so easily? The answer is actually the same for everyone. The answer is *accountability*.

Most people do not find the accountability they need to stay on track long enough to make a significant transformation. You need to do more than eat healthy and fast. You need to have an external accountability source to keep you on track. Let's return to the image of trying to carry a heavy, bulky couch up a flight of stairs all by yourself. You literally cannot do it alone. Nor can the strongest man you know. If weight loss has eluded you for months or years, then reaching your weight loss goal feels like carrying a heavy, bulky couch up a flight of stairs all by yourself. You cannot do it alone! You need a partner to carry half of your burden. You need someone holding the other end of the couch, carefully navigating each step with you, until you reach the glorious landing at the top. An external accountability source believes in you and already sees you as the future success-story version of yourself. They know you will make it to the top and will stay with you, carrying a half of your emotional load, until you get there. Studies show that yo*u will* get to the top, 95% of the time, when you have external accountability. Do not skip this step in your weight loss plan! Find a coach or a partner so that you will succeed.

You also need to commit to make the healthier decision in service of your highest good, *right now*. But how do you do that? How do you make the healthier decision when the BBQ chips are right in front of your face? There are a lot of different ways we do that. I will continue to give you the tools you need in order to transform into the healthier version of yourself, while we continue boosting your metabolism and burning your excess body fat with the SEXY Diet.

CELEBRATE YOUR WINS!

Here is a power tool to help you choose the healthier version of yourself. This tool is simple and fun. It's celebrating your wins. That's the tool. Celebrating!

If you do not take time to celebrate the little things along the way, then it is unlikely you will reach your ultimate goal, which is transforming into your future, success-story self.

Let's get started with celebrating all of your wins since you have started reading this book. What changes did you make in service of transforming into your future, success-story self? Did you create your future, success-story self? YES! That is awesome. Celebrate that win! Did you eat more vegetables? Yay! Celebrate that. Seriously, pat yourself on the back. Did you choose water over soda at any point this week or ditched the sugar in your coffee? That is a huge step. Congratulations! I seriously mean that.

I want you to take a few minutes right now to create a list of all of the changes you have made in service of your health and weight loss goals.

Congratulate yourself for each and every one of these big and little changes that you have made to becoming your future, success-story self!

Did you try fasting? I hope you are congratulating yourself right now if you did!

OK, if you are anything like me, the little voice is creeping in saying, "yeah, I tried fasting on Thursday, BUT I only made it to 3pm."

I want you to turn it around. There are no "buts" in celebrating your wins. You fasted until 3pm! That is so much longer than you have ever gone before! Celebrate that win. When you celebrate the little things, you open yourself up to more and more wins.

Circulate the energy of winning all around you by celebrating the small things. You need to do this every day, all day. Honor yourself for all of the good things you have been doing in service of transforming into your future, success-story self.

Celebrate the big wins too, but know that even the little wins are deserving of a big celebration. Take time today and every day to celebrate all of the positive changes you have made to improve your health and accelerate your fat loss. You have already begun to transform into your future, success-story version of yourself. Have a fabulous time celebrating yourself today and every day!

GRATITUDE

How do you find happiness in the present moment? One word: Gratitude. Perhaps you already have a gratitude practice in place. For those of you who are unfamiliar with gratitude as a spiritual practice, it is basically an intentional practice where you take a few minutes every day and look for things in your life to be thankful for. You may either write them down or take note in your mind of things around you that you are grateful for.

Gratitude is a game changer. If you do not already have an intentional gratitude practice, begin one today because this tool will help you transform into your ultimate success-story self.

How does gratitude transform you? Gratitude helps you discover happiness in the present moment. Like celebrating all of the little wins, gratitude circulates the energy of good things around you and helps you create more of the good stuff in your life, right now.

What are you grateful for right now? Quick, name ten things that you are grateful for in your life, right now. Find ten things in your life that you are authentically thankful for. Feel that thankfulness. What are you grateful for, right now, in this red-hot moment?

You do not need to spend very much time practicing gratitude every day for it to make a positive transformation in your life. You can do it in the line at the grocery store instead of being annoyed that the person in front of you is slowly writing a check, wasting your precious time. I love practicing gratitude in the car; beginning with feeling grateful for every green light or nice-looking car, or friendly driver, then moving on to all of the things about my family I am grateful for. You can do it while brushing your teeth, in the shower, or just take a couple of minutes after your meditation practice to intentionally give thanks for all of the good things in your life.

BLESS YOU

When you look around and see someone who has something that you really want, but you don't yet have, it is normal to feel the painful emotions of jealousy or envy.

"She's so skinny; I can't stand her".

"That rich guy is such an A-hole".

"She has the best wardrobe, I hate her for it!"
We have all had these feelings of envy and jealousy for others. It stems from our own insecurities that we will never actually achieve our own hopes and dreams. Envy and jealousy will hold you back from achieving your hopes and dreams.

The tool in your toolbox to combat this self-sabotaging habit is to send blessings to those who have achieved that which you desire to achieve. Even if they are a total a-hole, send them blessing on their way. Bless their totally undeserved trust fund. Bless their annoyingly fast metabolism. Bless their perfect hair, perfect spouse, and perfect body. Bless those who are driving around in your dream car and currently enjoying your dream vacation.

Get in the habit of blessing those who have what we really desire. You will transform into success-story version of yourself so much faster when you bless those who are already living it. Keep planting seeds of positivity, nourish and water them with love and the most beautiful flower you can imagine will bloom.

CHAPTER 15

Keto, Paleo, Plant-Based or the Mediterranean Diet?

WHAT'S BETTER? KETOGENTIC, PALEO, PLANT-BASED OR THE MEDITERRANEAN DIET?

One of the biggest questions I get asked all the time is, "what's the best diet: keto, paleo, vegan, or the Mediterranean Diet?" Here are the highlights of each of these diets so that you can understand the differences and possible benefits of each of these 4 popular diets and decide whether any of them are right for you. They are all compatible with the SEXY diet; you can choose to follow any of them, or skip this section if you just want to follow the guidelines of the SEXY diet.

The Ketogenic Diet

The Ketogenic Diet, otherwise known as keto, is a dietary plan where you limit your carbohydrate intake, eat low to moderate amounts of protein, while getting 75- 80% of your calories from healthy fats. The primary aim of the ketogenic diet is to put your body in a state of ketosis. Ketosis is achieved when you burn fat as your fuel source, rather than glucose. Glucose is the fuel source your body burns when you eat a higher carbohydrate diet.

Often confused with the Atkins diet, there are two main difference between the two. The Atkins diet does not discern between healthy and unhealthy fat, so people following the Atkins diet tend to consume a lot of saturated fat from animals. Keto focuses on healthy fats, such as extra virgin olive oil, coconut oil, butter sourced from grass-fed cows, and fats naturally found in plants, such as avocados, olives, nuts and seeds.

The other primary difference between keto and Atkins is that you must restrict protein to moderate levels in order to stay in ketosis, so the infamous bacon wrapped burgers of the Atkins diet are *not* keto compliant. When your body is in ketosis, it will convert any extra protein you eat into glucose, kicking you out of ketosis. It is just as important to limit protein intake as it is to limit carb intake to maintain ketosis.

While the ketogenic diet is known for being a high-fat diet, it is also a diet high in vegetables. You must restrict carbs to under 50 grams a day to achieve ketosis, however, nearly all of your carbs come from vegetables on a ketogenic diet. 50 grams of carbs may not sound like a lot, but in reality, you will eat more than 50 grams of carbs because the carb-restriction rule applies to *net-carbs*. This means you subtract the grams of fiber from the total carb count. Vegetables are very high in fiber, so when you subtract out all of the grams of fiber from the grams of carbs, you are left with a diet high in vegetables.

The ketogenic diet is not meant to be practiced indefinitely. Ketosis is a state to be practiced cyclically. Your body is designed to burn carbs as fuel just as much as it is designed to burn fat for fuel. Having the flexibility to switch back and forth between the two is the definition of metabolic flexibility. Metabolic flexibility appears to be one of the main benefits of practicing a cyclical ketogenic diet. The benefits of metabolic flexibility include a faster metabolism, mental clarity, increased insulin sensitivity and the ability to burn more fat when you are not exercising.

The ketogenic diet does emphasize eating a lot of healthy fats, but it also includes an abundance of healthy vegetables. The main thing people restrict on the ketogenic diet is sugar, processed foods, and protein. You can easily follow the SEXY diet and the Ketogenic diet at the same time.

The Paleolithic Diet

The Paleolithic Diet, otherwise known as Paleo, is modeled after what people imagine what our ancestors ate during the Paleolithic era. People have imagined it as a hunters and gatherers diet and typically eat lots of meat and veggies. Similar to the SEXY diet, sugar and processed foods are eliminated, which lends to the success that people have had with this diet.

The biggest concerns people have around the paleo diet is that people are eating way too much meat on this diet. It has become known as "the bacon" diet.

Some of the biggest advocates of the Paleo diet have more recently abandoned the paleo lifestyle and turned to the ketogenic diet, because they have found that the emphasis on protein has been more harmful than good. Other than that, many people have found success with this diet because it gets them back to eating real foods and completely cutting out processed foods. The Paleo diet is compatible with the SEXY diet.

The Plant-Based Diet

Also known as the vegan diet, the plant-based diet is a dietary lifestyle that excludes all animal products. The reason the name has shifted from vegan to plant-based is because the intention of following a vegan diet is to improve health while respecting the lives of animals. When the emphasis was previously just on avoiding animal products, many fell into the trap of eating a crappy diet, full of processed foods, such as crackers, bread and tons of vegetarian meat substitutes. Meat substitutes, such as veggie burgers, offer little to no nutritional value. A diet based on crackers and meat substitutes will destroy your health as fast as a poor diet involving animal products.

To avoid these pitfalls, the vegan diet has evolved into the plant-based diet, which emphasizes eating a diet high in plants, while eliminating all animal based foods. The plant-based diet can be an extremely healthy diet and there are decades worth of studies glorifying the health benefits of a plant-based diet. It is very compatible with the SEXY diet.

The Mediterranean Diet

Lastly, the Mediterranean Diet mimics that of the people living in one of the five blue zones, Sardinia,

Italy, as well as other parts of the Mediterranean. It is a diet that excludes refined sugar and flour, while emphasizing fresh vegetables, seasonal fruits, whole grains, nuts, wild seafood, and extra virgin olive oil. The Mediterranean Diet has been studied almost as much as the plant-based diet and is also celebrated for being heart healthy and for its weight loss benefits. It is compatible with the SEXY diet.

The SEXY Diet

As you can see, all four of the above popular diets all subscribe to the S in SEXY, which is, "sugar & flour free". They all subscribe to the E in SEXY, which is, "eat your veggies". And they all subscribe to the Y in SEXY, which is, "yes to healthy fats". They are all very different, but have some key similarities. None of them explicitly talk about the X in SEXY, which is, "eXtend your period of fasting". That said, one of the things that I love about fasting is that almost everyone can do it. You can fast if you are plant-based, paleo, keto or if you follow the Mediterranean diet. If you have a nut allergy, a dairy allergy, or a gluten intolerance, you can absolutely practice intermittent fasting. If you want to follow one of the above diets, you can still be SEXY.

Honestly, I really do not care which of these diets you subscribe to, as long as you are SEXY. Each of these dietary guidelines boast their own set of positive benefits. I feel like some people thrive on a plant-based diet while others do better practicing ketogenic cycling, while others still thrive on the Mediterranean style diet. Everyone has a different constitution. The good news is that you can follow the SEXY diet guidelines while on any of these diet plans, of following no other plan at all.

The SEXY Diet is actually not a diet. Diets do not work because anytime you cut calories, your metabolism slows down, unless you are fasting. Clinical studies have supported this again and again. The only safe way to cut calories, without slowing down your metabolism, is through fasting. The SEXY Diet is a lifestyle to include in whatever eating plan you subscribe to. It works for vegan's, Paleo, ketogenic, Mediterranean, gluten-free, or any other diet plan you may follow. Follow the SEXY diet for life and your metabolism will be fast and happy for life!

CHAPTER 16

The Enemy

EMOTIONAL EATING

One of the very first clients that I ever worked with was named Jessica. Like so many others, Jessica has a history of engaging in emotional eating. Jessica goes through a predictable cycle with her weight loss goals. She gets really excited about starting a new diet plan. She eats really well for four or five days, but then something happens and her anxiety gets triggered, and before she knows it, she is struggling to digest an entire container of cake frosting along with a super sized portion of guilt, shame, and self-hatred.

Sound familiar? One moment your inner health guru is in charge, making healthy, empowering choices all day, and then all of a sudden, you are lying on the cold, hard ground, succumbing to an urge to eat an enormous amount of your health sabotaging food of choice.

The food is often in your mouth faster than you can say, "HELP!" Anxiety and panic take you out of control and lead to emotional eating. Emotional eating is not a lifelong prison sentence and you do not need five-years of therapy to overcome it.

It is important to forgive yourself every time you succumb to emotional eating. Emotional eating is often not just emotional; it often has a biological component to it as well. Remember when I talked about authentic hunger versus hormonal induced hunger from sugar and flour? If you include sugar and processed foods in your diet, panicky hunger reactions are partially physical and harder to overcome.

YOU DON'T NEED FOOD, YOU NEED A HUG

If you suspect you are one of the millions of people labeled, "emotional eater", then allow me to break the news to you: you are not special. Most people have done it. Many people do it daily. You are not a bad person for having done it, and you are certainly not alone. That does not mean you should continue doing it though. If you are an emotional eater, it is helpful to ask yourself, "What am I trying to silence?" You carry layers of emotional beliefs that you have picked up throughout your life, beginning as a small child. It is not your fault. These stories and beliefs are a part of you and you may not even know they are there. These thoughts and beliefs are often lurking in the shadows of your mind, and trick you into believing they are facts. This is what makes emotional weight loss so challenging.

You may have a habit of eating cookies every time you feel sad, because your mother always fed you cookies when you felt sad as a little girl. Maybe your babysitter always gave you candy to shut you up when you threw a tantrum. Perhaps the first time your heart was broken, the only solace you could find was in a plate of french fries or an entire box of girl scout cookies, or both. Everybody carries different emotional connections with food. What I do know is that you don't *need* food when you are feeling *emo*. Food doesn't heal your emotions. It never has and it never will. What you really need is self-care, a hug, or some connection with nature.

EMOTIONAL DETOX

The truth is, at some point you are going to have to go on an emotional detox. You prepare for an emotional detox, not with green juice, but with a simple question, "what emotions am I suppressing with sugar and carbs?" The answer to this question will be your guide through your emotional cleanse. I don't know your story personally, but I do know that you have a unique story and that your story is a painful one. I have never met anyone who has not experienced a profound disappointment, sadness, injustice or traumatic event.

After four years of graduate school in psychology and many hours of clinical training, I have come to the realization that you do *not* need to go back into the past and ruffle up all of your old emotionally charged stories in order to heal from them. From the depths of my soul, I believe that you *can* work through your painful emotions by staying in the present moment and intending a rad future. Of course, there are exceptions. Exploring painful stories from your past in therapy can be helpful for some, but not everyone needs therapy to overcome emotional issues. When I say that you are going to have to address the emotions that you are suppressing with sugar and carbs, I don't mean that you are going to have to *relive* the stories attached to these emotions. This is not productive. You do, however, need to acknowledge them so that you can free yourself from the them.

This often looks a little something like this, "I'm craving an entire box of Oreo's right now. I wonder if there is an emotion underneath that? Oh yeah, my husband pissed me off this morning when he rolled his eyes at me when I couldn't decide what to wear. Why did he do that? Does he think I look fat in my clothes? Does he hate the way I dress? I hate when he rolls his eyes at me. I feel humiliated when he rolls his eyes at me. It reminds me when my mom used to roll her eyes at me when I was a little girl. I feel unloved when people roll their eyes at me. I want to eat a box of Oreo's instead of feeling unloved. Wait, I don't need an Oreo, I need my husband to not be a jerk. I need him to hug me, not roll his eyes at me." Or some sort of version of a story like that. Identifying the underlying emotion and story, then learning to ask for a hug, instead of reaching for a box of Oreo's, my friends, is harder than it sounds. At least in the beginning. It's like building a muscle. At first it feels really hard, but if you keep lifting those weights, or rather ask for a hug instead of a box of cookies, then it will get easier.

THE CRAPPY THOUGHTS WE FEED OUR MINDS

The most important phase of any detox is to stop exposing yourself to the toxins you are detoxing from. I have asked you to stop eating crappy food. I am now going to ask you to stop feeding your mind crappy thoughts. When you roll your eyes at yourself when you look in the mirror, you are feeding your mind crappy thoughts. When you throw shade at another woman who wears a size 2, you are feeding your mind crappy thoughts. When you throw shade at another woman who wears a size 22, you are feeding your mind crappy thoughts. When you throw shade at whatever size you are currently wearing these days, you are feeding your mind crappy thoughts. Throwing shade is a crappy habit. Practice throwing gratitude and acceptance instead.

Weight loss involves cutting the negative self-talk just as much as cutting the sugar. Stubborn thoughts will ravage your mind just as much as sugar will ravage your thighs. But just like you have probably been feeding your thighs some crappy food for years, you have been feeding your mind some crappy thoughts for years, if not decades. I do not recall every hearing of a successful weight loss transformation that did not involve an emotional transformation as well. You must work to lose your fears, guilt and shame along with losing the weight. Stop eating guilt, shame, and powerlessness with each bite, and instead, eat gratitude, joy and love with each meal. You do this by reaching into your toolbox and finding the right tool for *you*. Each tool works differently for everyone, but I encourage you to always begin by using your tool of visualization to get clear on what you *do* want. Then, reach for any of the other tools, all of which will help you gain freedom from hating your body while gaining freedom from your sugar and carb cravings.

Life is a journey, filled with ups, downs, and surprises at nearly every turn. It is messy, beautiful, smelly, exhilarating, terrifying and hilarious. Seriously, all six of those things happened this morning while I was getting my sons ready for school. Every day is a journey and many of the days on my journey, my emotional baggage gets dumped right in front of me. I used to strive for perfection, but I have learned that perfection is the wicked step-sister of control. It has taken years, but I have finally learned that I am not in control of what happens here on planet earth. The only thing I can control is the way I respond to the mayhem around me. As I continue to release the emotional baggage I have picked up along my life path, I feel freer and lighter. My body weight reflects this. I work at it daily, and invite you to do the same.

When your emotional detox has taken a bumpy detour and you have found yourself stuck at the side of the road in a state of panic, sometimes shoving food down your throat is the only solution you can think of. I want you to consider grabbing for this new, shiny power tool to fix your car, instead. The best tool I know to overcome the panic associated with emotional eating is a tool called *tapping*. It is time to put this awesome tool into your toolbox of successful weight loss!

TAPPING

I am going to take you through a brief introduction to the Emotional Freedom Technique (EFT), otherwise known as "tapping". If this tool feels like something you would like to utilize on a regular basis, I encourage you to research it further. There are countless free resources all over the internet. I have personally watched several Youtube videos with great tapping scripts that can help you overcome the panic and anxiety that cause emotional eating.

Typically, you begin tapping by identifying your stressful trigger on a ten-scale. So, on a scale from 1-10, how freakin' badly do you want that candy bar. Rate it. If its anywhere from a seven to a ten, then tapping is going to be a great tool for you to reach for.

Have you ever seen a karate master break a brick block with their bare hand? In my son's karate studio, they say, "Hai!" The edge of their hand that they break the brick with is where we begin tapping. It's called the karate chop point. With the tips of your fingers from your other hand, you tap the karate chop points while saying, either out loud or in your mind,

"Even though I freakin' want the candy bar so bad right now, I love and accept myself."

Repeat it three times. And if candy bars aren't your jam, insert whichever food is your biggest weakness.

"Even though I want the freakin' chips and salsa so bad right now, I love and accept myself."

"Even though I want to eat the entire tub of frosting so bad right now, I love and accept myself."

Then you move to the other points. Just keep reading and keep tapping along. You tap each point six or seven times, it doesn't really matter how many times, just keep tapping while talking.

The next point is the eyebrow point. Tap, tap, tap the inside of your eyebrow while saying, "This craving is so intense!"

Then move to the outer eye. You can either choose one side or do them both. It doesn't matter. Tap the outer eye while saying, "I want it so bad it hurts."

Move to under the eye. Tap under the eye while saying, "I am going to explode if you don't shove the entire candy bar in my mouth right now!"

Now begin tapping above the lip, under the nose while saying, "I don't think I can handle getting through another minute without eating this candy bar."

The next tapping point is the middle of the chin, under the lip. Tap, tap, tap while saying, "the only thing that can possibly make me feel better, is this candy bar."

Move down to your collar bone. Tap right under the collar bone while saying, "I need to fill myself with this candy bar right now."

The next tapping point is underneath the armpit, at your bra line. Tap here several times while saying, "I can't handle this anymore."

Then move to the top of your head and tap there several times while saying, "I can't go much longer without shoving a candy bar down my throat right now!"

Then repeat the sequence, skipping the karate chop, over and over again, until you begin to feel some emotional release. Soon, the intensity of your craving with dissipate to a more manageable level.

WHY TAPPING WORKS

The tapping points are based on your body's natural energy meridians and each tapping point is connected to your emotional body. Tapping works similarly to acupuncture. In acupuncture, the needle is the tool used to move energy, whereas in tapping, you send energy through the meridian just by tapping on it, so that your body can heal naturally. Tapping moves stuck energy, so the emotions are released, rather than trapped in your body. And it works!

It is too hard to manage a craving when your craving is at a nine on a ten scale. We have all been there before! The plate of cookies is right in front of you; you are hungry and dying for one of those cookies! They are as good as in your belly when your craving is at a nine. But if you can get it to a four, you can make a healthier decision much more easily. Tap when your cravings are at a nine and see if you can stop yourself from making a decision you will soon regret!

Back to tapping:

Keep going through the tapping points, saying whatever comes up, such as, "I need this right now".

"I can't live without this candy bar."

"I feel like I'm going to die if I don't eat this candy bar right now."

Go through all of the tapping points until you feel some emotional freedom. Once you are there, feel free to tap in some positive affirmations.

POSITIVE AFFIRMATIONS

"I've got this".

"A candy bar is not what I need right now; I need a hug and I'm going to go get me one!"

"I forgive myself."

"I can choose a healthier food."

"My future-self is so proud of me for making a healthier decision!"

"I love myself."

"I choose health."

"I am safe; I am loved."
Play with this for a bit today and decide if a tapping practice is right for you. It can be a very powerful tool in your tool box. Get ready to lose the emotional baggage you carry around and joyfully express your confident, healthier, thinner self.

CHAPTER 17

The Very Ugly Shadow

My team was recently redoing my website and they wanted to have more before and after pictures of me on the BodySoulShine website. Specifically, they needed more *before* pictures. We had enough pictures of *skinny Summer* but they wanted more *before* shots to illustrate my transformation.

So I went into my iPhoto's and searched and searched but I couldn't find any. Every picture of myself that I had personally saved during the several years that I lived in a heavier body did not show my heavier body.

Without realizing it, years had gone by where I had basically deleted every picture of myself that showed my overweight body. I found quite a few pictures where I had cropped my body out of the shot, so I had tons of super close up pictures of my puffier face, but virtually none of my body. I had to snag the *before picture* that I am using on my website from my sister's Facebook page. I remember being so mad at her for posting that picture, because I was so ashamed of how overweight I looked, but I am now grateful because it is one of the only pictures I have of my full body during the several year period that I lived in a heavier body.

This was actually a big surprise because I don't remember making a conscious decision one day to delete pictures of my body, it just sort of happened.

SHAME STEALS YEARS FROM YOUR LIFE

Shame and self-hatred can be very sneaky; we often fail to realize that they are driving our car, steering us away from our goals. I felt too much shame to even look at my body, so I got rid of any pictures of it without even realizing it. I am sharing this today because I suspect I am not alone.

In fact, I know I am not. I have another client, Shannon, who avoided taking any pictures of her body as well. She told me a heartbreaking story when we first started working together. Her mother so badly wanted a family portrait with her adult children to hang on the mantle. For years, Shannon's mom had begged her to do a family portrait and for years, Shannon told her mom that she would do it when she finally lost the weight.

Year after year went by and Shannon never lost the weight. Year after year went by and Shannon's mom was denied her wish of having a picture with her beloved family to look at and cherish every day.

Shannon's mom got breast cancer and after a couple years battling cancer, it became clear that she wasn't going to live much longer. She finally convinced Shannon to do the family portrait. Sadly, Shannon's mom died before she actually saw the final product. The photographer wasn't able to get the pictures to the family until after her mother had died.

Shannon's profound body shame prevented her mom from getting her dream of having a nice picture with her family. Shannon *always* thought that she would one day lose the weight and give her mother the gift of the family portrait. But year after year went by and the weight never came off.

Shannon now has the family picture with her deceased mother hanging in *her* home. She has lost weight since the picture was taken and lets the photo motivate her to continue on her weight loss journey.

HOW IS YOUR EXCESS BODY WEIGHT HOLDING YOU BACK?

What I want to know is, how many other people out there are avoiding family portraits?
How is your excess body weight holding you back? Do you avoid having your picture taken? What else are you avoiding? The camera is not the only thing that we hide from when we have excess body weight. I have personally witnessed several people avoid going for job promotions because they don't feel that they are good enough because of the way they look. Many people hold themselves back from going for a career advancement because their weight has stripped their self-confidence. This is heartbreaking.

I wish it was not true, but for most women, our self-confidence is directly tied to our body weight. It shouldn't be, but it is. Our body weight does not just affect our health and energy levels. It affects our romantic relationships, finances, where we choose to go on our vacations, and whether we buy nice clothes for ourselves. Our weight can affect our friendships, our relationship with ourselves and even our relationship with god. It doesn't have to be this way. Shame does not have to dominate your life.

THE TOLL SHAME TOOK ON MY BODY

For years I was unable to lose the weight because I was crippled by the shame of living in an overweight body. I really hated myself because I had been thin for many years and in a short 2-year period of time I put on 30 stubborn pounds that I could not exercise off my body. I was following the horrible weight loss advice to "diet and exercise" and the scale was my constant enemy.

I was stuck in the frustrating pattern of yo-yo dieting, characterized by exciting weight loss, followed by the inevitable weight loss plateau, and finally culminating in the regaining of all of my weight back. The crappy cherry on top of this awful yo-yo dieting pattern is that I was stuck with a slower metabolism, despite the fact that I was exercising more than I had ever exercised in my life.

I remember feeling scared because I had to exercise *a lot* and cut calories, just to maintain an overweight body. I was feeling much more than just shame, I was also feeling despair because I believed that if I stopped exercising so much, I was going to get even heavier. I was in a lot of pain because my body isn't supposed to exercise that much, because I have hip dysplasia. I cannot exercise as much as most healthy adults without causing a flare-up to my hip; flare-ups are painful, so I was in a ton of pain from over-exercising and eating the wrong kinds of food.

Yoga Pants & Bathing Suit Cover-Ups

The shame held me back from so much during this time. I avoided doing anything that would have required me to wear anything other than yoga pants. Cocktail parties, swimming pools and nice dinners with my love were virtually absent from my life. It is embarrassing to say this but I would find excuses to say no to going to certain parties and events because I did not want to have to wear a bathing suit in public, or a cocktail dress in front of other thin women.

I went to Hawaii once during the time I was heavy, but I only brought one tankini, and wore it only during the couple of times that I went snorkeling. Otherwise, I covered my entire body in these 'cover-ups' that I had spent *so* much money on. The bathing suit cover up was way more important than the bathing suit itself.

My shame stole years worth of pictures of me and my husband. I avoided the camera like the plague. I felt inadequate at work, because of my weight, even though my weight had nothing to do with my job. I let my body weight determine my self-worth.

MY MOST EMBARRASSING STORY

What shame does to you is it takes away your rationality. One of my most embarrassing stories was a direct result of feeling shame around my body weight. After 20 hours of labor with my first son, I gave in, and begged for an epidural. I know I am not alone in this one! When the anesthesiologist finally came into the room, he asked how much I weighed. Between contractions, I literally yelled at him, "look it up in my chart!"

I was not willing to say out loud how much I weighed, because I weighed more than my husband, and I was humiliated by the number. I did not want my husband to know that I weighed 200 pounds, even though there was an 8 ½ pound baby in my belly. Shame can make you think crazy thoughts and do crazy things! Shame prevented me from making rational decisions that fuel good choices. When shame rules your life, you do not go for your dream job, nor do you put yourself out there to go on a first date. You say, "no" to the party for fear of looking bad in a dress. You do not go on your dream vacation. When you are drowning in shame, you do not believe you can ever change, so you don't even try. Shame holds you back from living your full life and achieving your dreams, including your weight loss dreams.

You weight does not determine your self-worth. I love helping women find their self-confidence during the weight loss journey, not once they have achieved their weight loss goals, because the truth is we are lovable and worthy at any weight. Do not let shame take that away from you.

3 Easy Steps to Ditch Body Shame & Build Self-Confidence

Step 1: Acknowledge It

Do not do what I did. Do not let several more years go by where you avoid the camera. Bring awareness to your shame. Acknowledge your self-hatred, if that is what is going on for you. Acknowledge where your body weight is holding you back. This is not going to make the shame go away, but it is the first step you must take to make sure you do not live this way for more years to come. Be radically honest with yourself when you look at the hard stuff. You might be surprised to find that it is a relief to finally acknowledge how much your excess body weight has been holding you back.

Step 2: Set Intentions

Set your intentions to make powerful change. Be bold. Be brave. Let your secret day dreams become your intentions for change. If you secretly dream of confidently wearing a bikini, even though you've had five children, then let that secret fantasy become your intention. It does not matter how many children you have had or if you are in menopause, or if you think you have a freakishly slow metabolism, or whatever the story is in your head. These are just excuses that are holding you back. If you have a dream, allow it to become an intention, which will eventually become your reality, if you continue to take action toward making it come true.

The future, success-story version of yourself is likely the intention you will be setting. Intend that this version of yourself will manifest. Celebrate this and never lose sight of your dreams. Vow to make your dream come true each and every day.

Step 3: Take Bold Action, Now

You must take action, now, in this red-hot moment, so that you can turn this dream into a reality. Not tomorrow. It does not matter what the action is, as long as you do something. Now. Throw away the soda in the fridge, right now. Make three big salads so that you have healthy lunches for the next three days. Text your BFF and promise her that you are going to lose one pound this week and ask her to text you every day to check on your progress. There are endless possibilities. Choose one and do it right now. I believe in you! You've got this!

CHAPTER 18

Does Stress Really Make You Fat?

YES, STRESS REALLY MAKES YOU FAT

The clinical studies do not lie. Stress really does make you gain weight. Stress makes your body release the hormone cortisol, and cortisol forces your body to pack on the pounds. Stress also causes you to make poor food choices. Whatever the reason, every clinical study that looks at stress and body weight shows that stress makes you gain weight.

You undoubtedly have stress in your life. I do not know one person who doesn't have stress in their life. It is literally everywhere. Whether on the news, in your bank account, at work, with your kids, in your bedroom, or staring at you in the mirror, stress is lurking in every corner. Stress will always be a part of your life, but it is important to have daily practices that combat against stress. You often cannot change the external situations that cause the stress, but you can change how you respond to your stress. Let me repeat that. You do not have control of the vast majority of the external stressful things in your life.

But you have 100% control of how these external things affect you.

ACCEPTANCE

First you need to accept the things that are happening around you. Accept that they are happening and you cannot change them, so freaking out about them is not going to help. What *is* going to help, is to reach for your tools. Your tool box is overflowing with tools and practices that will keep your head above the water when stress is threatening to drown you. Reach inside your tool box and discover two new power tools inside!

BREATHE IN THE AIR

The first shiny new tool I am gifting you today is your breath. That's right, your breath. Most people breathe just to stay alive, but you can use your breath to combat stress. In fact, using your breath is one of the most powerful, yet simple tools to burn through stress.

Let's breathe together now, shall we?

Breath Technique 1: Inhale 1-2-3, Exhale 1-2-3-4-5

This simple breathing technique requires that you inhale through your nose to the count of three and exhale to the count of five. Do this five to ten times in a row, and it will instantly calm you down. The reason why this simple breathing technique of inhaling through the nose to the count of three and exhaling to the count of five works so well is because when you are stressed out, your sympathetic nervous system is activated. That's your "fight or flight" reaction. When your exhale is longer than your inhale, it instantly takes you out of the fight or flight state and puts you into your "rest and relaxation" state.

It has been described to me this way: the only stress our ancestors used to have was the stress of running away from predators. When your distant ancestor was running for her life, away from a saber-toothed tiger, she was desperately gasping for air, inhaling as much air as possible through her mouth. This put her in a sympathetic state, which was beneficial to help her run faster and survive. Survival is the only reason why anyone would want to be in a sympathetic, fight or flight state.

Sadly, modern day humans live in a perpetual sympathetic, fight or flight state, where we are constantly stressed out, as if we were always being chased by a saber-toothed tiger. There are literally no benefits to living this way. In fact, living in a constant state of stress is killing us. It is crucial to learn how to turn off your sympathetic nervous system and turn on your parasympathetic nervous system so that you can decrease your stress levels. You can do this effectively with a simple breath technique.

When you slow your breath down, inhaling through your nose to the count of three, and extend your exhale a little bit longer than your inhalation, you literally turn *off* your sympathetic nervous system and turn *on* your parasympathetic nervous system. That means you turn off our body's stress system and turn on your body's natural, relaxation system.

You cannot be stressed when your parasympathetic nervous system is activated. When you inhale through your nose to the count of three, and extend your exhale a little longer, to the count of five, you are sending signals throughout your body that force it to chill out and relax. Your body cannot stay in a panic when you breathe this way. You can calm your stress just by shifting your breath for as little as 30 seconds. It can be *that* simple.

Breath Technique 2: Square Breathing

This simple technique involves inhaling through your nose to the count of four, holding your breath to the count of four, exhaling to the count of four, and holding your breath again to the count of four. Try this for two minutes. This will calm you down and give you a sense of peace. It is a great way to relax right before going to bed!

MEDITATION FOR THE WIN

The other stress-busting power tool I want you to put in your tool box is Meditation. I am trained in Vipassana mediation, which is a simple practice of quieting the mind and gently focusing on your breath. I am also trained in Transcendental Meditation (TM), which is a form of meditation where you gently repeat a mantra in your head over and over again. In fact, I have tried several different forms of meditation throughout the years because I was kind of obsessed with finding the *right* form of meditation. What I have learned is that there is no right or wrong form of meditation. Sometimes I follow my breath, sometimes I return to my mantra, sometimes I listen to music to focus on, and other times I listen to fancy brainwave entrainment programs. They all work. They are all great. One is not right and none of them are wrong.

I know this because they all provide me a calming presence when I practice them regularly. When I am meditating regularly, no matter which form, I am able to manage my stress with ease. It is not magical; the neuroscientists have identified clear differences in the brains of regular meditators. Certain areas of the meditators brains are bigger, which is why they can manage stress more easily. Meditation is a practice that works when done daily.

JUST DO IT, REGULARLY

In order to address the stress in your life, I encourage you to use the breathing techniques regularly. Either choose square breathing or the technique where you inhale through your nose to the count of three and exhale to the count of five. I also encourage you to cultivate a meditation practice in your life. Meditation has saved me. I honestly think I would have physically harmed my mother in law at one time if it was not for my meditation practice. Meditation truly helps me stay calm in the face of stress. Instead of reacting to a situation out of stress and overwhelm, I am able to respond with clarity. I am able to respond with my chosen personality, rather than my *tyrannical toddler*, or any of my other multiple sabotaging personalities.

BAD NEWS/GOOD NEWS

Sometimes the news really gets me down. When terrible things happen in the world around us this does not mean that we need to break all of our weight-loss goals. During times of political stress, natural disasters and tragedies, you do not need to go back to the old ways of abusing your body. You will respond much better to external stressors when you are healthy.

If you find yourself eating a lot of foods that are sabotaging your weight loss goals, like kibble and Miracle-Gro, then the first step is self-love, no matter what. You cannot drag yourself through shame and self-hatred.

How do you achieve self-love and self-acceptance when you are under a lot of stress? First, normalize what is going on. Nearly everyone falls off the wagon at times. You are still loved and worthy, even when you are not loving yourself.

Stress can literally take the blood away from the parts of your brain that are in charge of your willpower, and feed the part that deals with survival. When you are in survival mode, you can regress to the behavior of eating everything in sight. This is actually a normal response when you are in survival mode. You will absolutely be able to get back to having stronger willpower when you decrease your stress levels.

DECREASE YOUR STRESS

How can you lower your stress if breathing and meditation aren't your thing? Even a simple 15-minute walk can make a significant impact on lowering your stress. Another one of my favorite ways to turn around a stressful day is to text one of my best girlfriends and tell them what I love about them. Try it! Make their day and see what happens. Spoiler alert: your stress instantly melts away, leaving a huge smile on your face in its wake.

In fact, finding five things that you are grateful for right now can completely destress you. Close your eyes, inhale through your nose, exhale through your mouth and list five things you are grateful for.

You cannot control the news cycle. School shootings, natural disasters, offensive politicians, and mean people are not going to go away. The only thing you can control is how you respond to these things. Shoving cookies in your face is not going help. Kindness and gratitude *will* help though. Making compassionate choices for your body will help keep you strong, focused, and of course, sexy.

CHAPTER 19

Detox Your Kitchen, Detox Your Thoughts

DETOX YOUR KITCHEN

If you haven't already, it is time to detox your kitchen. That means get rid of the foods containing sugar, flour, and polyunsaturated vegetable oils. Basically, all of the foods that come in a convenient package should be removed so you are not tempted to eat them. When following the SEXY diet, we replace these foods with nutrient dense alternatives. This likely means more work for you because you are going to have to do some cooking and meal prep.

THE POWER OF MEAL PREP

Once again, the super smart scientists are our best teachers. They have done a ton of studies about this and the conclusion they keep coming to is that those who take a few minutes each week to formulate a meal plan will be way more successful in achieving their health goals than those who do not formulate a meal plan.

Luckily for you, you do not have to be a scientist to get in the habit of planning out your meals each week. The SEXY Diet will work for everyone. If you are drawn to following the Mediterranean diet, you can do so while following the SEXY diet. The same goes for those who follow a plant-based diet, a ketogenic diet, a Paleolithic style diet, gluten-free, dairy-free or nut-free. You just need to leave out the sugar and flour, plan a couple of fasting days, and include an abundance of veggies with healthy fats at each meal.

BIG STEAMED POT OF VEGETABLES

My biggest secret to making sure I get enough vegetables in my diet is what I call my *big steamed pot of vegetables*. Twice a week I either go to the farmers market or the grocery store and buy a ton of vegetables. Broccoli, cauliflower, asparagus, brussels spouts, squash, kale, swiss chard, collard greens, spinach, those kinds of vegetables. I rinse them, cut them up, and steam them. All of them. I make a big pot of vegetables. Then I dress them with coconut oil or grass-fed butter, or whatever healthy fat I am in the mood for, put them in a couple of glassware containers, store them in the fridge, and my family is good to go on veggies for several days. Since they are already prepared, I easily reach for them with every meal.

I toss a huge handful of steamed veggies into my soup. The warmed broth instantly reheats the veggies and I get all of the nutrients and fiber my body craves. I mix veggies in everything. If I make spaghetti and meatballs for my family, I put the marinara sauce and meatballs over a huge handful of veggies, instead of over a heaping pile of pasta. I mix a heaping serving of vegetables in my lentils, quinoa, or on the side with a couple of eggs, instead of toast. My meals do not always look like the conventional meal that we are used to. I have learned to think outside of the box and put my veggies first.

I have learned the hard way that if I skip this step of preparing my big steamed pot of vegetables, then I make poor eating decisions. If my family wants burger night, I can order a grass-fed burger with a lettuce wrap, skip the fries and eat a large portion of veggies from my already prepared, big steamed pot of vegetables. Burger night has suddenly transformed into a healthy meal. If my family wants pizza night, they can enjoy all the pizza they want while I easily prepare myself a quick meal, filled with vegetables. Sometimes I will even enjoy a slice of pizza with them but I will also include a ton of veggies to fill my belly, so I don't stuff myself with four slices pizza, like I used to. When the veggies are already prepared, you will eat them.

DETOX YOUR THOUGHTS

After you detox your kitchen, it is time to detox your thoughts. I have a client named Angela who was not able to make a breakthrough with her weight loss goals until she detoxed her thoughts.

After beginning intermittent fasting, life started getting in the way of her goals. Angela had originally committed to fasting on Mondays and Wednesdays, but sometimes stuff would come up that challenged her resolve to abstain from food until dinnertime.

Meeting with a client, or a lunch meeting at work began to pose problems for her because Angela didn't want to make anyone feel uncomfortable with the fact that she was not eating. So instead of sticking with her commitment to fasting, Angela would break her fast and have lunch with her team members.

I challenged this belief that Angela had. I explained to Angela that it was her *belief* that told her that others would be uncomfortable if she wasn't eating lunch with them at the meeting; it was her belief, not a reality.

I asked her if she was sure that the others would be uncomfortable with the fact that she was not eating. I also asked her if they would really even notice and care? Angela thought about this and committed to going to the following Wednesday team member lunch meeting, and not touch any food. She was expecting to have to explain herself to everyone as to why she was not eating. But nobody asked. Nobody even seemed to notice that Angela was not eating. People are often so wrapped up in their own worlds, that they are not paying as close attention to you as you might think.

That was Angela's first win. A couple weeks later, Angela was going to a potluck style baby shower and was dreading having to eat all of the unhealthy, albeit tasty dishes provided, because she knew they would sabotage her health and weight loss efforts.

She thought it would be rude if she didn't eat at the party and she was scared people would think she was weird if she did not eat. That is crazy. But I love Angela, so I didn't tell her that she was crazy. I did, however, gently nudge her to realize it was her *belief* that others would think she was weird and rude for not eating at a party. I am so proud of her because she decided to fast on the day of the baby shower. She drank sparkling water and enjoyed the company of others. Nobody threw her shade. Nobody gave her side-eye. Nobody thought she was weird or rude. It was a monumental win for her; a huge breakthrough in Angela's life. She now feels empowered to go to parties and not eat if she does not want to.

THE 3 SECRETS OF HOW YOU ARE GOING TO BE YOUR GREATEST SUCCESS STORY

Secret 1: Cut the Sugar

Obviously, the number one reason why you are going to lose the weight is because of your willingness to decrease your sugar intake, beginning now. By now you know that you cannot exercise the weight off when you are eating sugar and flour.

One of my specialties is helping women titrate down, little by little, the amount of sugar and processed carbohydrates they are eating every day. It is hard to quit sugar cold turkey. It is physically hard, emotionally hard and psychologically hard. If it was easy, we would all stop eating sugar right now. But there is a reason why there are way more sugar addicts than cocaine addicts out there. Sugar really is addictive. That said, it is very possible to quit the sugar habit, especially if you have adequate support.

Secret 2: The SEXY Diet

The second reason why you *are* going to lose the weight is because you are going to follow all 4-steps of the SEXY diet and use your power tools of successful weight loss. I created the SEXY diet because every great system that has ever been invented is simple and accessible for anybody to follow. After reading literally dozens of books and articles from doctors, scientists and weight loss experts, I was able to distill down everything I learned into four simple, yet effective, weight loss principles. These four powerful weight loss steps will change your life. When you also use the power tools provided throughout the book to keep on track, you will transform your body and your life.

Secret 3: External Accountability

The third reason why you are going to successfully lose the weight…drum roll please…is *external accountability*. I know I am starting to sound like a broken record with this accountability stuff, but it is literally the most important thing that you are going to do to ensure your success. You cannot carry a heavy, bulky couch up a flight of stairs by yourself. If you have fantasized about meeting your weight loss goals for years, and feel like you have tried everything, but you've failed, then achieving your ideal body weight is as daunting as carrying a couch up a flight of stairs all by yourself. You need external accountability. You need a partner to take some of the heavy load off of you. You need a partner to balance you, guide you and keep you on track, reminding you to take one step at a time. I cannot stress enough just how profoundly important external accountability is on your journey.

You need to find an accountability partner or a program that offers you daily, external accountability to keep you on track. Studies show that when people set out to achieve a goal, they have a

25% chance success rate, but if you have a weekly external accountability source, you have a whopping 95% success rate. Enlisting an accountability partner or joining a support group can make all the difference for you. I would be honored to be a part of your accountability team. If you are looking for external accountability, go to my website, bodysoulshine.com for all of my offerings and find out the best way I can support you and hold you accountable to your health and weight loss goals. Whatever you do, find the accountability you need to reach the finish line. You will lose the weight and keep it off, because you are not going to let shame cripple you. You are not going to let sugar fuel you. And you are not going to let accountability slip away. You've got this, girl!

CHAPTER 20

How to Stay Healthy While Eating Out

SOCIAL SABOTAGE

My client, Lori was recently telling me that after having been so proud of herself for having lost several pounds and choosing foods that made her feel great, she sabotaged it all. And she kept repeating this pattern of going a few weeks of eating really well and losing weight, but then her social calendar would fill up and she would not keep to a healthy lifestyle. She would lose a few pounds and then put all the weight back on again. I have a pretty active social calendar and I manage to maintain my weight, so I was not going to let her off that easy. But it is worth a conversation because she is not the only one in this boat.

What really struck me is that she told me a story about drinking wine, even though she didn't feel like drinking wine. Her two closest girlfriends texted her to meet them at an impromptu girl's night and before she knew it, she was applying mascara and lip gloss and rushing off to their favorite restaurant before happy hour was over. But she wasn't in the mood for happy hour food and wine. She had spent the entire week making empowered decision after empowered decision in service of her weight loss goals. The success-story version of herself had been in the driver's seat all week long, until her friends texted her, then her inner party girl jumped in the driver's seat and whisked her away to happy hour.

THE DREADED IN-LAW'S

I have another client, Shannon, who was dreading going to dinner at her in-law's house because she felt she had to eat everything her mother-in-law prepared, because she did not want to offend her mother-in-law. She didn't want to be rude, so she ate every single thing her mother-in-law made, including the homemade apple pie for dessert, even though she doesn't even like apple pie.

Ladies, why do we sabotage our own health and weight loss goals in order to avoid offending others? Is it really so offensive to put your own health and weight loss goals above other people's feelings? That is a question I would like you to ponder the next time you find yourself at someone else's house faced with eating something they made, that you do not want to eat. Is a simple, "no, thank you" really that offensive?

More likely than not, people are not even noticing what you are eating. And most good people will not be offended if you skip their homemade dessert because you are currently engaged in a weight loss program. Most people will be inspired by your resolve to put your health first.

Are there other areas in your life where you put other people's feelings before your own? Are you making health-sabotaging decisions so as not to offend somebody else? I want you to ask yourself the following question, "why do I care so much about what they think?" Then weigh your answer against how badly you want to achieve your ideal body weight. Which is more important to you?

When was the last time you did this? I can tell you I've done it more recently than I would care to admit. Why do we sacrifice our own health and weight loss goals for fear of missing out? Why can't we find a way to socialize with our friends that does not involve self-sabotage?

I want to challenge you to put your health first from this day forward. I want you to be *offended* by the thought of putting somebody else's feelings before your own health. Your health and weight loss goals come first, girlfriend. Take a stand for yourself. Dare to love yourself enough to say "no, thank you".

I came up with a 5-part plan for Lori. Here is how Lori stopped sabotaging her weight loss goals in 5 easy steps:

STEP 1: IT'S ALL IN YOUR HEAD

Most mother-in-laws are not terrible. They are not going to hate you if you don't eat their apple pie! Most of them have also tried to lose weight at some point in their lives, so they totally know what you are going through. Assuming that they will be offended that you don't want to eat their homemade pie is all in your head.

I had Lori call her mother-in-law prior to their next dinner to let her know of her weight loss goals and that she would not be indulging in dessert until she had reached her ideal body weight. Guess what, her mother-in-law made a super healthy dinner! See, not all mother-in-law's are terrible!

STEP 2: PISS OTHER PEOPLE OFF

If your mother-in-law *is* terrible, or the person you are having dinner with is super judgy, then let them be terrible and judgy. It is OK to piss people off sometimes and not eat their homemade dessert. It is OK to say, "no, thank you" to food that does not fit into your eating plan. If they get mad, that is a reflection of them, not you. This is such a great opportunity for you to practice being OK with not pleasing others! Your health comes first!

STEP 3: PRE-EAT

Pre-eat if you know dinner is going to be super unhealthy. Or bring your own food! Honestly, I have done both. I usually pre-eat and then eat the veggies at the dinner.

STEP 4: VEGGIE OBSESSED

When you are at a restaurant, order a double portion of veggies, instead of the potatoes and veggies. Also, avoid the bread. My family recently vacationed in Hawaii and we ate out at restaurants five nights while we were there. At each of the restaurants, my husband and I ordered both appetizers and entrees, but we ordered our appetizers from the *side dish* menu. It seemed like every restaurant had these awesome brussels sprouts side dishes, so we got the brussels sprouts as an appetizer a few times, to ensure we were getting tons of veggies because I am obsessed with vegetables. We actually got broccoli as an appetizer one night, and it was some of the best broccoli I have ever tasted. Every dinner was awesome. We ate tons of good food with lots of veggies.

Plus, it is way more fun to run around on the beach in a bikini the day after eating broccoli and brussels sprouts than the day after gorging on flat bread and fried calamari. Am I right?

STEP 5: GOOD FRIENDS

This one is so important. Surround yourself with friends and family who totally love and accept you and support your goals. My girlfriends do not judge me when I say, "no, thank you" to a cocktail at girl's night. My girlfriends also do not judge me when I *do* decide to eat a cupcake or have an extra cocktail. And they do not judge me when I *don't* eat these things. This is probably because I don't judge them when they make these decisions for themselves. Step five is really just about kindness and love. Love yourself. Love your friends. Let's stop judging ourselves and stop judging our friends and support one another. That, my friends, is the best one I've got for you.

INDULGE IN YOUR FAVORITE FOODS WITHOUT GAINING WEIGHT

It *is* possible to indulge in your favorite foods sometimes and continue to lose weight. How often? That is the Million Dollar question. It is time to have a reality check about this, because there are a lot of special occasions that fill up our social calendars, and it is not reasonable to indulge at all of them and think you will still lose weight. Whether the occasion is date night with your love, ladies' night with your girlfriends, or any number of the year-round holiday parties that we participate in, it seems like every time we go out, we are indulging in food and drinks that we know are going to sabotage our health and weight goals. How much do you associate socializing with food?

THE CYCLE OF LIFE

There are holidays nearly every month of the year that involve massive indulgences, many of which we do not want to miss out on. In February, Valentine's Day is filled with chocolate, candy, and wine. March brings us beer & fatty foods at St. Paddy's Day. Then comes Easter, which is another major sugar-fest. The season of summer brings us tons of BBQ's and picnics, all of which involve carb heavy foods, cheese, wine and other sweet treats, at least where I live, out here in Wine Country! Then the fall arrives, which means we are inundated with everything pumpkin spice. Like everything, from pumpkin spice lattes to pumpkin spice muffins and pumpkin spice oatmeal. Which leads us into the peppermint and eggnog season. Then the calendar year turns over and we do it all again.

We are connected to food throughout each of the holidays and special occasions on an emotional level because food hits all of our senses, which further connects us to these holidays. Many foods that we eat on special occasions smell amazing, they taste like their corresponding holiday and they even look like the holiday's. Sweet treats with holiday inspired flavors have begun to symbolize each of the holidays for us in so many ways. They emotionally connect us with all of our senses and we feel drawn to indulge in all of these special treats, whether they be cookies, or latte's, savory meals or sweet treats. Food around each holiday or special occasion carries a deep emotional connection for us.

THE URGENCY TO INDULGE

To add fuel to the fire, you only get to have these things once a year, so it creates a frenzy and urgency to indulge in all of your favorite treats because they are not going to be available to you again for an entire year. Each holiday only comes once a year. My husbands' birthday only comes once a year, my oldest son's birthday only comes once a year, my youngest son's birthday only comes once a year, and on and on and on. By the end of the year, we have had so many birthdays, holidays, anniversaries, girl's nights and special events, all of which are filled with weight-sabotaging foods and beverages.

Each time there is a special occasion, the little voice comes into your head, telling you that it is OK to indulge this time, because you can just go on a diet once the holiday is over. The little voice tells you that it is a special occasion, so you *have* to indulge! This little voice tells you that you will just start eating clean again on Monday. Have you ever told yourself that one?

This is where I want to invite you to pause for a moment, girlfriend. A reality check is in order. The holidays and birthdays and special events add up in a year. Once you are done with one, there is another one right around the corner. Always!

If you are trying to lose weight or just to maintain your weight right now, special events and holidays do not have to be the enemy. You just cannot let all of them be an indulgence fest. I do not believe in 100% deprivation. I advocate a "cheat meal" every week during weight loss, so you do not feel deprived.

HOW TO ENJOY IT ALL WITHOUT GAINING WEIGHT

Do you want to know how to enjoy all of your favorite special occasions and holiday treats when you are trying to lose weight or even maintain your weight? Good. Here we go.

Step 1: Delay Breakfast

On the day you will be indulging at a special event or holiday party, delay your breakfast. Then, have a really filling late lunch. I would suggest eating a ton veggies and healthy fats with a moderate amount of protein, which will keep you full. I love eating my signature fat salad on days I know I will be indulging at an evening event. The point is to not show up hungry. You can indulge in your favorite foods, just don't eat unreasonably large quantities.

If you find yourself going to more than one special event in a week, always swap a carb heavy meal for an ultra-healthy one, filled with vegetables, healthy fats, olives, avocado and a moderate amount of protein.

Step 2: Drink Lots of Water

I know you have heard this one a million times before, but it is worth a reminder because it is so important. If you are drinking alcohol, ALWAYS drink a glass of water between every alcoholic beverage! Don't forget to do this! It will slow you down, preventing both hangovers and embarrassing behavior.

Step 3: Limit it to just One

If its pumpkin spice season, do *not* have a pumpkin spice latte every flippin' day. If you look forward to these things all year long, like so many of my girlfriends do, make it a special occasion that you get to enjoy *one*. Do not enjoy 12 of them this year when pumpkin spice season rolls around! Those specialty drinks have so much more sugar in them than you can imagine.

Sadly, not only is sugar super addictive, but it makes you super hungry. The worst thing you can do is drop a bunch sugar in your body day after day. This is just going to make it harder to wean yourself off of the sugar when you finally make the decision to lose your unwanted body fat. Keep it to one specialty beverage during the holiday season!

I am not going to sugar-coat it for you: Sugar really is the enemy! You can enjoy sugar on occasion, but if you include it in your daily diet, then it becomes a problem. Feel free to indulge in your favorite sugar-bomb treat a few times a year, just do not indulge in them daily or even weekly if you are trying to lose weight!

Step 4: Share the Love

Don't make the mistake I used to make every December! My mother-in-law makes Russian Tea Cakes every year at Christmas time. This is an heirloom recipe she received from her mother who likely received it from her mother. These cookies are amazing and they are literally my favorite treat when the holidays roll around. When I was a heavier gal, before I had lost my weight, when my mother-in-law would bring a tin full of these cookies, I would gorge on them. I would eat like 7 or 8 of them, possibly more. I would eat them until I felt sick, and then, every day after that, I would let myself eat 3 Russian Tea Cakes a day until we ran out.

That is not a good game plan, my friends. I absolutely do not encourage this behavior with your favorite annual holiday treats! Instead, do what I do *now*. Now, when my mother-in-law brings over a big tin of my beloved Russian Tea Cakes, I let myself truly enjoy a couple of them, and then pass the rest along. Share your treats with someone who is not concerned with their weight. Do not hoard them for yourself. I really recommend allowing yourself to mindfully enjoy a nice treat once a month or maybe twice a month, depending on your weight loss goals. Mindfully means being present when you smell it and taste it and really allow yourself to enjoy it. Do not eat until you feel sick, you know?

Step 5: Avoid Sugar

I know I talked about this in Step 3, but I need to make sure I get the message across, so it's in Step 5 as well. Hear me out: the less sugar you eat, the less you will crave it. And you will really enjoy those special occasions so much more when you do indulge, if you indulge only once or twice a month. It can be helpful to remember that eating sugar is like spraying Miracle-Gro on your fat cells. It can also be helpful to equate eating sugar with eating kibble. Who wants to think of dog food when they are eating? Gross.

USE YOUR FAVORITE CHEAT FOOD TO LOSE WEIGHT

I had a client named Jenny who brilliantly used her cheat food to lose all of her unwanted weight. When we first started working together, Jenny told it to me straight: there was no way she would ever be able to go an entire day without eating a fudge popsicle. She was dead serious; she could not make it through one day without her beloved Fudgsicle. It literally got her through the day.

This posed a problem for me, considering how much sugar those things are laced with. Jenny had some serious weight loss goals and I had a serious objective to get the sugar out of her diet. She was able to give up all other forms of excess sugar, except for her Fudgsicles.

I was admittedly annoyed at first. "Really?" I thought. "You *really* can't go one flippin' day without a Fudgsicle?"

But the truth is, knowing that she could eat her one Fudgsicle every day gave Jenny the strength and willpower to knock out all of the soda, granola bars, and bread she was eating. She eliminated a lot of the kibble in her diet, just by allowing herself to have one Fudgsicle a day.

Months went by and the pounds *were* slipping off of her, despite her daily Fudgsicle. Let me tell you, I know *my* body well and if I ate a Fudgsicle every single day, I would start to put on some weight. Everyone has a different metabolism. Jenny's body was responding really well because she was actually eating way better than she ever had before because instead of eating a daily granola bar, sandwich, soda and a Fudgsicle, she was now only eating a Fudgsicle, along with a ton of other healthy veggies, fat and protein.

Without any nagging from me, one day Jenny told me that she had gone three days without eating any Fudgsicles. She needed her Fudgsicle crutch for several months to help her titrate down from all of the other excess junk, but after a while Jenny finally gained the confidence to go a day without any cheats. She went three days. Now Jenny eats only a couple Fudgsicles a week, and she is at her ideal body weight!

Use your crutch food to your advantage. Allow yourself your one beloved treat food each day for a while, as long as everything else is squeaky clean. Then one day, see if you can drop it. Titrating down off of sugar can be so much easier than going cold turkey.

FAIL YOUR WAY TO THE FINISH LINE

The wise sages remind us that failure is temporary. They remind us that failure is our great teacher and without failure, we cannot learn and grow. Failure is never a destination, and it is one of the most important parts of your journey.

If you have failed to get to your ideal body weight, then please learn from this. Look at it this way, if you have a physical injury, your doctor will treat you and monitor your healing progress. If you are not getting better your doctor, or physical therapist will accept that the treatment is not working and try something different.

The same needs to be applied to your weight loss and weight maintenance plan. If you are stuck in a weight loss plateau, meaning the scale has not budged in several weeks despite your efforts to make it budge, then you need to try a new strategy, because what you are doing is not working.

Also, I know that weight loss plateaus are the most frustrating thing on planet earth. So, it is totally OK to feel super frustrated, angry and sad, but you have to give yourself a time-limit for these feelings! Otherwise, they will take over and sabotage your weight loss success. So, feel the frustrating feelings, but only for like an hour. Never let yourself stew in negative feelings for more than a day! Clock in to your pity-party, then clock out. You have to shift it. You *can* shift it and you *have to* shift it, so that you will achieve your greatest success.

How do you shift out of your pity-party? There are very powerful, yet simple ways to do this. The best way to shift out of a pity-party is to ask yourself, "What am I grateful for right now?" and force yourself to answer that question five times. Find five things that you are grateful for. Then, ask yourself, "what am I proud of myself for?" Again, answer that question five times. Find five things that you are proud of. Then, finally, finish this sentence, "Today I am choosing to be…"

Hopefully your answer will involve choosing to change your weight loss strategy to one that is going to rock your world! Choose to be the empowered version of yourself. Choose to operate from your success-story version of yourself. Choose to put the healthier version of yourself in the driver's seat.

SUCCESS IS NOT YOUR DESTINATION

Just like failure is not a destination, success is not a destination either. You will always strive for success. You strive to meet your goal, but when you get there, you find that it too is only a temporary place in your never-ending journey.

You grow from both places; you grow from both failure and success. They are both equally important. It is not the destination that will bring you your greatest happiness, it's the journey! Am I right?

What I want you to focus on during your journey is progress. Progress is what you are always looking for on any journey. Celebrate your progress, each and every day.

Were you a failure this week at meeting your weight loss goals? Or were you a model of success? Either way, I commend you for being awesome! Both are great and both are very temporary. Look for what is working and strive for progress.

What progress are you celebrating right now? I know that I am really proud that I have maintained my ideal body since having both of my children! I am celebrating the fact that I am healthier in my 40's than I have ever been in my life.

I am a huge advocate of celebrating your successes! Throw yourself a party for all of the little things, just don't get yourself a cake. I recently asked my client, Sara, to identify ten little successes that she was proud of for having accomplished in the past week. She found 26. That kind of blew my mind. What successes can you celebrate right now? I bet there are a lot more than you think.

What failures can you celebrate? What I mean is, what failures are your growing through? The wise sage was not born a wise sage. Let your failures birth your wisdom and become your ultimate successes. Keep celebrating those failures, those successes, and most of all, celebrate the progress you are making along the way, my friends. Enjoy the journey. That is what sets us apart from the rest and will ensure that you will become the success-story version of yourself.

CHAPTER 21

Lose Fat, Gain Pleasure

SUGAR IS NOT SO SWEET, AFTER ALL

We consume 20 times more sugar now than our ancestors did. Sugar is toxic to our livers at this quantity and is making us very sick and quite frankly fat. I do not want to spend more time talking about the evils of sugar though. I have done that enough in this book already. You get it. I know. I do, however, want to talk to you on a personal level about how ditching sugar has completely changed my life.

I was born with hip dysplasia. You might have an elderly canine friend who suffers from this painful condition. I have known several dogs who have hip dysplasia, and when I watch them limp around, unable to jump or run anymore, I want to cry. I truly feel their pain. Hip dysplasia can be pretty awful.

I am lucky though, because my hip dysplasia is milder than some. It didn't affect me until around my 30th birthday, which is around the time I started gaining weight. When my painful symptoms began, I thought I had injured myself jogging. For years I suffered tremendous pain in my right hip, and I thought it was from a jogging injury. I would be fine for a few days or and then all of a sudden, I would get these flare-ups out of nowhere. These painful flare-ups in my hip made walking, sitting, and even standing hurt. I couldn't even think about exercising.

I am telling you this because the orthopedic doctor who diagnosed me told me that I would have to take strong, prescription strength anti-inflammatories for the rest of my life in order to control my pain.

I spent several months wondering why anti-inflammatories worked to make my pain level go down. I mean, what was causing this inflammation anyway? Since inflammation was causing my pain, not the hip dysplasia itself, was there a way to avoid inflammation, rather than treat it with a pharmaceutical drug? I wondered, was there a connection between my diet and my inflammation?

THE INFLAMMATION CONNECTION

Sure enough, when I stopped eating sugar and processed foods, my pain literally vanished! Cutting out sugar and processed foods has been the best thing I have ever done in my life, besides getting married and having children, of course! Since I have stopped eating sugar and processed foods regularly, I have not had one significant flare-up of my hip dysplasia pain.

Yes, I lost over 30 pounds, which probably helped relieve the pressure on my hip. But I go days on end where I literally forget that I even have hip dysplasia. If I sit for too long or exercise too hard, I am reminded of my hip issue. But I do not walk around in massive pain any more.

Even though the orthopedic doctor told me that I would have to take prescription strength anti-inflammatories for the rest of my life, I don't take anything for pain, because I do not have any pain anymore. I no longer need anti-inflammatories, because my body is no longer inflamed. My body is no longer inflamed because I no longer eat kibble.

If weight loss is not a big enough motivator for you to change your diet, then maybe pain will be your motivator. Cut out sugar and processed foods for one week and replace them with veggies and healthy fats and watch your pain melt away.

DO ARTIFICIAL SWEETENERS MAKE YOU FAT?

Artificial sweeteners are everywhere, from diet soda, to Splenda in your coffee, NutraSweet in your tea, and sucralose in your protein powder. What's the big deal about artificial sweeteners? They have no calories, so they must be good for weight loss, right? The answer might surprise you. Studies have come out that artificial sweeteners are strongly correlated with weight gain.

Some clinicians say that artificial sweeteners increase your insulin levels, even though they don't have calories, which is why they cause weight gain. Other doctors say that the inflammation artificial sweeteners cause is what prevents you from losing weight. Still others have suggested that artificial sweeteners desensitize your taste buds to the sweetness that is naturally found in whole foods, which sabotages your enjoyment of healthy foods. All three are likely true.

Whatever the case, diet sodas and artificial sweeteners are very strongly associated with weight gain, and should be removed from your diet when trying to lose weight.

Soda and diet sodas are not only implicated in weight gain. There are also clinical studies showing that they are associated with a shorter life span and a higher risk for stroke and dementia. If weight gain is not a strong enough reason for ditching sodas and artificial sweeteners, then dementia, stroke and premature death surely are.

If you have a soda habit, you are not alone! About half of all Americans drink soda daily. It can be challenging to quit cold turkey, but it is absolutely possible to kick the soda habit.

YOUR CHALLENGE, IF YOU CHOOSE TO ACCEPT IT

If you drink several sodas a day, I want to challenge you, right now, to cut down to only one a day. If you are only at one a day right now, then your challenge is to quit cold turkey. You can do it. Yes you can, you sexy beast!

You might find it easier to replace soda with sparkling water garnished with a wedge of citrus. Some prefer unsweetened iced tea or just plain old-fashioned water. Whatever your preference, find a healthy replacement. Your body and metabolism will love you for it!

REALITY CHECK

When making big changes in your life to lose weight, you want the weight loss to happen fast. Here you are, engaged in a whole new weight loss system, making some profound changes in your life. You are eating a lot of vegetables, you are abstaining from food at times, you are likely cooking more, perhaps with different ingredients than you are used to. I want to applaud you for making all of these health-promoting changes in your life.

I also want to acknowledge that typical results for any weight loss program are one to two pounds a week. When you have 20, 50, or 100 pounds to lose, one to two pounds does not feel like a lot for all of the effort you have put in. Just remember, days can feel long, but weeks and months fly by. Think about it, every year when the holiday season rolls around, you are always in shock, wondering where the year went. A year is not that long. If you keep working the SEXY weight loss system, you are going to transform into your future, success-story version of yourself before you know it. Keep up the good work, every day. This time next year, your future self is going to be thanking you so hard!

It can be challenging, I know. This is why you need to frequently connect with your desired outcome. You need to stay connected to your future success-story version of yourself and have her be your biggest cheerleader. Ultimately, she is the one that is celebrating each and every healthy decision you make.

FOLLOW YOUR GUT

I am now going to shift the weight loss conversation to one of my favorite things to talk about, which is the gut microbiome. Your gut microbiome refers to the community of trillions of bacteria currently living in your gut. There really are trillions of little guys colonizing your body right now. You have way more bacteria living inside of you than you have cells in our body. For every tiny cell in your body, you have ten bacteria, which is a lot.

We have been conditioned to believe that bacteria are bad, but we could not survive without these guys. It turns out, these bacteria help you thrive; they help you digest your food, they can speed up or slow down your metabolism and help regulate many of your bodily processes.

Interestingly, the bacteria that you have are largely determined by the foods you eat. And guess what? Good bacteria, the ones that promote health, including a healthy body weight, eat healthy foods. Guess what kind of food bad bacteria like? You probably guessed it: sugar and processed foods. If you eat lots of food that comes in a package, you know the ones: the ones that are filled with sugar, processed flours and vegetable oils, the ones that ultimately cause inflammation, well, it turns out, bacteria that thrive on these kinds of foods are shown to be abundant in people with health problems, such as type 2 diabetes, obesity, inflammatory diseases, heart disease, digestive problems and even cancer.

Scientists are starting to see a correlation between the healthy food that we feed our bacteria, and our overall health. You can dramatically change your own health by doing three simple things. You need to eat fermented foods, prebiotic foods, many of which are found in vegetables, and reduce or eliminate sugar and processed foods from your diet.

FERMENTED FOODS

Fermented foods contain probiotics. The probiotic works kind of like the military, protecting you from foreign invaders otherwise known as bad bacteria. Prebiotic foods, on the other hand, actually feed the good bacteria, so these colonies grow. You really want to grow your colonies of good bacteria, so include prebiotic foods in your diet regularly. Onions, garlic, jicama, asparagus, dandelion greens are some of my favorite prebiotic veggies. Another classification of prebiotic foods is called resistance starch. Foods high in resistant starch are resistant to digestion, which is actually a good thing because while *we* do not digest them, they are actually used as food for certain good bacteria in your gut.

And then, this is actually kind of funny, the poop, for a lack of a better term, or maybe we should just call it the *waste* that these bacteria create, is actually food for the cells that line your intestinal wall. These cells need to eat too, and when they eat the waste from the good bacteria, your gut gets to be super healthy and happy. The cells that line your gut walls need you to eat prebiotic foods so they can eat too. Ideally you will eat prebiotic foods in your diet every day to keep your gut healthy and happy.

HOW TO STOP SUGAR & CARB CRAVINGS

The other really cool thing about your gut bacteria is that it plays a crucial role in your cravings. When the colonies of bad bacteria are greater in number than the colonies of good bacteria, your cravings for the kind of foods that are going to feed the bad bacteria are greater as well. But once you consciously shift your diet and feed the good bacteria, while starving out your bad bacteria, your cravings will change.

I cannot tell you the last time I ate chips and salsa, which was one of my major food cravings for years. I used to get intense cravings for them and eat an enormous pile of salty chips with sugary salsa until I would feel sick to my stomach. I literally do not crave chips and salsa anymore, and I used to crave them almost every day.

Chocolate chip cookies were another one of my weaknesses. I would frequently find an excuse to bake them and eat a ton of cookie dough followed by several warm baked cookies. I never even think to make them anymore. I eat a chocolate chip cookie with my sons once or twice a year, but more often than not, when I am at the bakery buying them a cookie, I easily pass without any desire or discipline. I do not feel tempted to steal bites from them because I do not crave that kind of food anymore.

Do you want to know what I *do* crave? Broccoli. I'm totally serious! I often crave avocados mixed with sauerkraut, as well as steamed kale with grass-fed butter. I cannot go a day without veggies because I literally crave them. How cool is that? Now is the time to begin including prebiotic and probiotic foods in your diet so that you can stop craving sugar and carbs and start craving foods that will turn on your skinny genes! Your digestion will improve, your cravings will change and your energy levels will soar!

GET PLEASURE FROM SOURCES OTHER THAN FOOD

Pleasure is an important part of life. You are likely used to getting a lot of pleasure from the food you eat, which is normal and healthy. But far too often food becomes the primary source of pleasure in peoples lives. It is important to focus on gaining pleasure from sources other than food while on a weight loss journey. Of course, it is absolutely acceptable and expected that you will continue to let food be a source of pleasure, just don't let it be your only source of pleasure.

What comes to mind when we talk about pleasure? Sex of course!!! Sex is one of the biggest sources of physical pleasure you will ever experience. Let's dive right in to how you can intensify your physical pleasure during sex, so you do not have to rely on food for all of our pleasure.

There are huge differences between men and women when it comes to arousal and pleasure through sex. We have to talk about this huge elephant in the room. I am totally going to freak you out right now and talk about porn. That is totally not what you were expecting me to say, right? Don't worry, I am definitely not advocating you go watch porn or anything like that! The subject of pornography is a great place to start because it so clearly shows the difference between how men and women experience pleasure.

I am sure most of you have not, but if you have ever watched a pornography film, you know when a man has achieved an orgasm; he cannot fake it. Men do not have the ability to fake their orgasm like Meg Ryan did in "When Harry Met Sally."

Here is the crucial difference between men and women: Every woman that has ever performed in any pornographic film, is faking it. 100% of the time. How can I be 100% confident of this, considering that I am not a porn star nor have I ever been involved in the pornography industry? I am absolutely confident of this because it is not physically possible for a woman to achieve an orgasm unless she has one very important thing: the hormone Oxytocin.

OXYTOCIN

Oxytocin is actually the hormone that women experience when they are breastfeeding. It is known as the love and bonding hormone. It is the hormone we produce when we are lovingly connecting with our loved ones. I promise you, no porn star has ever received a rush of oxytocin on a porn set. OK, enough about porn. I am definitely not an advocate of pornography. In fact, I despise the pornography industry because it has ruined countless lives. From porn addiction (a very real and serious issue) to the countless women forced into sex slavery via the porn industry, and several other disturbing issues, I am not a fan of pornography. I am simply using pornography as an example to illustrate a point that women have different needs than men when it comes to pleasure.

Let's bring this back to you; assuming you aren't a porn star (I am so wishing that I could insert a bunch of silly emoji's in this book right here!). In all seriousness now, what I want for you is to increase more oxytocin in your primary love relationship, if you are currently in one. The more oxytocin you have, the more pleasure you will be able to experience in the bedroom in your monogamous, loving relationship.

Notice how I said, "monogamous". Yes, this is true. Women need to feel safe, loved, respected, cared for and understood to make oxytocin. If you are not making enough oxytocin, then you will not be able to achieve physical pleasure. This is one of the stronger arguments for humans being monogamous, at least for *female* humans. Men do not need oxytocin to achieve physical pleasure, only women do.

SYMBIOTIC RELATIONSHIP

How do you increase your oxytocin levels naturally so that you can increase pleasure? You do this via a symbiotic relationship with your love partner. You cannot nag your husband/partner to make you feel safe. You cannot nag them to make you feel loved and cared about. You cannot demand that they respect you.

You must evoke these feelings out of your partner by giving him what he needs. Relationships work best when there is a balance of giving and receiving. According to the New York Times bestselling author, and psychologist John Gray, in a heterosexual relationship, men need to receive appreciation, trust and acceptance. Let me repeat that: Men *need* to feel appreciated, trusted and accepted for who they are. These three feelings increase their testosterone levels, which decrease their stress levels. There are clinical studies to prove this! When men feel appreciated, trusted and accepted, their stress levels go down. When their stress levels go down, they have more energy to meet their partner's needs. I love symbiosis!

The more *your* needs are met, the more you have to give to your partner. The more your partners' needs are met, the more he has to give to you. It is a true, symbiotic relationship. If you are in a heterosexual, monogamous relationship, then practice giving your partner what he needs, so that you inspire him to give you what you truly need: more caring, understanding, and respect. When you get more caring, understanding, and respect, your oxytocin goes up, making you feel happier, more loved, and you get lots more *pleasure.*

You can reach your ideal body weight by giving your partner more of what makes him feel good: appreciation, trust, and acceptance. He, in turn, will give you more caring, understanding and respect. It is a win-win because everyone experiences more pleasure in the bedroom, and the icing on the cake is that when we experience more pleasure in the bedroom, we also avoid late night snacking. The benefits are endless!

OMG I cannot believe I talked about porn in this book! That was crazy! I hope it was helpful though. Following the SEXY diet is the foundation of achieving your weight loss goals. Attending to the needs of your primary relationships will also help you cross the finish line. I hope you will try this out and give your partner more appreciation, trust and acceptance, if your partner is a man, or more caring, understanding and respect if your partner is a woman. Attending to these primary emotional needs to your spouse/partner is another powerful tool in your toolbox of successful weight loss.

CHAPTER 22

Your Overflowing Tool Box

TOOL BOX REVIEW

It is time to review all of the sexy, shiny tools you have in your tool box for successful weight loss to make sure you are using them. The first four tools in your tool box are your *Master Tools*! These four tools, the 4-part weight loss system known as the SEXY diet, are the most powerful tools you have to shrink your fat cells, speed up your metabolism and turn on your skinny genes. The remaining tools in your tool box are your Power Tools, and they will give you the inspiration, drive and accountability to stay on track and meet all of your goals.

Let's review them and make sure you are incorporating all of these master tools and power tools into your life.

MASTER TOOLS

1. The **S** in SEXY stands for, "Sugar & Flour Free"

2. The **E** in SEXY stands for, "Eat an Abundant of Vegetables"

3. The **X** in SEXY stands for, "eXtend Your Period of Fasting." This tool will not only help speed up your metabolism, but it is the most efficient tool you have to melt the pounds away.

4. The **Y** in SEXY stands for, "Yes to Healthy Fats"

POWER TOOLS

1. **Visualization:** Specifically, you regularly visualize your future, success-story version of yourself. This is you, who has achieved all of your hopes and dreams. This personality is real. It lives in the future, but loves visiting you daily to give you inspiration and encouragement.

2. **Choose wisely:** You have multiple personalities; the tool is to *choose* which personality to put in your driver's seat. Ultimately, you want to choose the success story version of yourself most of the time.

3. **Spiritual guidance:** You have an external spiritual helper guiding you and divinely helping you; whether it be Jesus, an angel, the Universe or a deceased relative; you are getting spiritual support to keep you on track.

4. **Time-Restricted Eating:** You practice time-restricted eating, which means you begin eating at the same time every day and you stop eating at the same time every day. Ideally, you are eating in a six to eight-hour window every day and you do not eat anything once

your window has closed, not even a single blueberry.

5. **Polyphenols:** You eat lots of polyphenols every day to turn your skinny genes on! You choose organic whenever possible, because organic foods have way more polyphenols in them.

6. **Know your multiple personalities:** You have the tool of identifying other health-sabotaging personalities that take over the driver's seat, such as your *tyrannical toddler* and *inner hot mess.* After you identify the health-sabotaging personalities, you choose a health-promoting personality.

7. **Self-love:** Self-love is a tool that I hope you reach for daily. It is important for you to know how to discern between self-love and self-sabotage and to cultivate deeper self-love every day.

8. **Tapping:** You have the tool of Tapping to decrease your anxiety and panic, so you can *choose* to remove the tyrannical toddler from your driver's seat, and replace him with a much better driver.

9. **The Cycle of Life:** When pumpkin-spice season rolls around, you limit it to just one pumpkin spice treat, rather than one-a-day. There are special occasions around each corner. Indulge in some and abstain during others.

10. **Water:** When you feel hunger, you reach for a glass of water first, because thirst is often mistaken for hunger.

11. **The Power of Positivity:** You know that your mind and body are connected and a

slight shift in your thoughts can have a powerful shift in your body. Your tool is to plant seeds of positivity and choose your thoughts wisely.

12. **Intentions:** You set powerful intentions each day, each week, and each month so that you know what your goals are. Stay connected with these goals daily.

13. **The Power of Now:** You take action, NOW, in this red-hot moment, toward meeting your goals and intentions.

14. **Breathe:** Breathing is a simple yet profoundly useful tool. You practice square-breathing or you inhale through your nose to the count of 3 and exhale on the count of 5 whenever you feel stressed out.

15. **Meditation:** This is a phenomenal stress reliever and life-transforming practice, if practiced daily.

16. **Celebrate:** You celebrate all of your big and little wins every single day. You make loads of positive, healthy choices every day, and you celebrate each and every one of them!

17. **Gratitude:** Your gratitude practice circulates more happiness in the present moment. Gratitude helps you create happiness both in the present and the future.

18. **Bless You:** When you look around and see someone who has something that you really want, but don't yet have, instead of getting crazy with jealously, you have cultivated the habit of blessing those who have what you desire. You will transform into success-story version of yourself so much faster when you bless those who are already living it.

19. **Meal Prep:** You pre-prepare healthy meals to take to work, such as salads; and you steam a big pot of vegetables twice weekly to ensure you are always including an abundance of vegetables in your diet.
20. **Heal your gut:** Eating fermented vegetables can dramatically improve your gut health make you stop craving Kibble-like foods, which spray Miracle-Gro on your fat cells.
21. **Exercise:** You do not exercise for weight loss because you know that exercise does not lead to weight loss. You exercise for your health, never for weight loss!
22. **Pleasure:** You know how to get pleasure from sources other than food!
23. **Cheat Meals:** You use your cheat meal to your advantage.
24. **Artificial Sweeteners:** You haven't only ditched sugar, but you have also ditched artificial sweeteners.
25. **Share the Love:** You share the love, gifting all of this knowledge you have gained, because if you want something, you give it.
26. **Open your tool box daily:** You reach into your shiny, sexy tool box each and every day!

That was 30 SEXY Master Tools and Power Tools that you currently have in your shiny tool box for successful weight loss. Make sure you are taking these tools out regularly to sculpt, chisel, and craft the healthiest, most glorious version of yourself that you can imagine.

CHAPTER 23

Synchronicity Revisited

COINCIDENCE VS SYNCHRONICITY

Some people do not believe in synchronicity and feel more comfortable using the word coincidence. These people are missing out on receiving an amazing gift. Coincidences do happen and are more common than synchronicities. Randomly running into the same person twice in one day in two different places can be called a coincidence. A synchronicity is much bigger than a coincidence. A synchronicity is a profound coincidence that is life affirming. Synchronicities feels like the hand of God has moved mountains to create a series of wonderful events. When it feels as though external forces are working in your favor to create something wonderful for you, it can no longer be called a coincidence, it has gone into the realm of synchronicity. Synchronicity has an element of magic to it, and always brings deeper, spiritual meaning. In some cases, synchronicities change lives.

Do you remember the story I told you in the chapter entitled, "Synchronicity", about my mother during the time she was going through cancer treatment at UCSF? It is a personal story that illustrates the undeniable difference between coincidence and synchronicity. I told this same story of my mother's life-affirming synchronicity with the man from UCSF at her memorial service in 2005. Back then, I thought the story had ended at the music festival in Mendocino with the musician from UCSF, but little did I know, the synchronicities continued long after my mother's death. And my life will never be the same.

MY MOTHER'S GIFT TO ME

The oncologist at UCSF recommended that my mother go into Hospice care so that she would remain comfortable in her final days. Words fail to describe how soul crushing it was for me to watch my mother make a decision to transition from fighting for her life to accepting death. She had fought cancer for 17 years, and was considered a medical miracle up until that point. I secretly thought my mother would always be the miracle story that inspired countless other cancer survivors. She wasn't supposed to die. She was supposed to live forever to prove that miracles *do* happen. Little did I know, the miracles would continue after her death.

My sister and I both took a leave of absence from our jobs and moved in with my mother and our step-father during her last month of life. It was a blessing to spend every last day with her, as if to drink every bit of her in, knowing she would soon be gone forever.

Looking back on this time, my sister and I frequently say, "I don't know what we would have done without Hospice." Hospice expertly cared for all of my mother's challenging and ever-changing physical needs, so that we could attend to all of our emotional and spiritual needs. My mother's Hospice nurse, Linda, was a guiding light through what was the darkest days of our lives.

After my mother's death, I knew I wanted to give back to this wonderful organization that had given my family more than we could every thank them for. Linda, our hospice nurse extraordinaire, referred me to the hospice volunteer program, where I participated in a 6-week program to become a hospice volunteer. To my surprise, Linda showed up with flowers to the graduation ceremony when I completed my training. She then recommended that I serve my very first official hospice volunteer placement to a patient she was then working with.

I had temporarily moved in with my step-father to help with the aftermath of my mother's passing. Linda noted that the woman I would be caring for lived just around the corner from my home.

For the next three months, every Tuesday, I would walk over to my neighbor's home and serve as a volunteer to help the dying woman and her bereaved husband. I had never met these people before, but cultivated a lovely connection with them. They were an elderly couple who both carried advanced degrees and appreciated the company of a younger graduate student. I enjoyed my Tuesdays with them, even though it was relatively brief. After the woman died, I moved on to working with other people in Hospice, and mostly lost contact with Gary, the widower who lived around the corner.

This was a darker time of my life. I had ended a toxic relationship shortly before my mother's death and was now living in a town with few friends, overwhelmed by my grief over the loss of my mother coupled with the stress of graduate school. I desperately wanted to get married and have children, but couldn't even find a man to go on a date with. Months went by and I questioned whether I would ever have the opportunity to have children. I made a pact with God on New Year's Day of 2007. I promised I would be open to meeting new people in hopes of finally meeting my soul mate.

Within two weeks, out of the blue, I received a phone call from Gary, the elderly widower who lived around the corner. I hadn't heard from Gary in months! He told me that he wanted to introduce me to the man who lived next door to him. He explained that his neighbor was a friendly, single man and thought we would, "hit it off".

I was absolutely horrified at the thought of being set-up by my elderly neighbor, but I had literally made a pact between myself, God and the Universe, less than two weeks before this phone call, to say *yes* to dating. Because I couldn't go back on my word with God, I was unable to say, "no, thank you" to Gary's friendly offer, even though I felt humiliated by the thought of being set up by a senior citizen who barely knew me. I reluctantly agreed to walk over to his home later that week, for an informal meeting between neighbors.

Over a decade later, my husband and I love telling the story of how our crazy neighbor, Gary, set us up on that fateful night. We both have different versions of how we each dreaded going to this man's house to awkwardly meet another single person, and both did so out of obligation. We were both pleasantly surprised to have been set up with a very attractive person and couldn't wait to get out of

Gary's house so we could get to know each other in private.

The thing is, Gary is the last person you would have expected to have set us up. He was the most hated man on our street. Other neighbors held decades-long grudges against him. He had no friends. He had anger management issues and he tended to drink too much. But Greg and I were the only two young people that Gary knew at the time and we were both kind to him, so he set us up. Had Gary not introduced Greg and I, we never would have met and our sons, Jude and Skyler, would not be alive today.

SYNCHRONICITIES KEEP ON GIVING

I feel the hand of God in this story of how I met my husband. I also feel my mother expertly orchestrating the details, as she often did in life. How can it be just a coincidence that my mother's hospice nurse led me to the man who would later introduce me to the father of my children?

Synchronicities are blanketed with magic and blessings. Synchronicities are life-affirming and keep giving life. Had any of these events not occurred, my beautiful children would not be alive today. Every detail is woven together in a perfect fabric of synchronicity. Beginning with my mother's UCSF experiences, leading to the hospice nurse, my conviction to volunteer my time for this organization and getting placed with Gary, culminating in Gary feeling inspired to introduce the only two young people he knew, all of these events are a deep blessing in my life that have brought me my husband and two children. Had one of these things not happened, I would never have met my husband, Greg, despite the fact that he lived right around the corner from me. I believe in the power of synchronicity and I offer gratitude to this power daily.

Many parts of the story happened *to me*, but I also took action that helped move the synchronicity along. I had a strong intuition that I needed to volunteer for hospice, and despite my own overwhelm and grief, I entered into the hospice volunteer program. Despite feeling strapped for time as I balanced graduate school, a job, and my grief process, I committed to volunteer 3 hours of my time each week. I took action based on a gut feeling, which helped move the synchronicity forward. Likewise, I had set an intention to get married and have children, despite not having any dating prospects around. I opened myself to the possibility and promised God that I would say yes to any dating opportunity that came my way. I did not turn my back on this promise and was rewarded handsomely when I did say yes.

SYNCHRONICITIES ALL AROUND

My parting words to you *begin* with this image of synchronicity. Synchronicity is not a tool you can put in your tool box of successful weight loss. Synchronicity is a gift that comes from beyond. You must invite synchronicities into your life by listening to your deepest desires, set clear intentions to turn these desires into reality, and then say *yes* to opportunities! Take inspired action! You must know what you want and move toward your goals with conviction and a willingness to try new things. I strongly believe that without even knowing it, you are in the middle of a synchronicity right now. You set an intention to lose weight and were somehow guided to *this* book. Watch for life-affirming signs. Follow your intuition. Say an enthusiastic *yes* to new experiences and possibilities. Keep taking inspired action and offer gratitude to all of the interesting twists and turns you find along your path.

YOU ARE A BLESSING

My parting words to you *end* with the same words I spoke to you at the beginning of this book. You are God's greatest gift. Experiencing a human life on this magnificent, blue planet is the highest honor and greatest gift given to you. You are a soul of great importance. You are a gorgeously unique expression of this creative energy we call God or the Universe. There is no better expression of gratitude for your life than by living it to the fullest, continually moving toward your wildest dreams and saying yes to opportunities and experiences. May this book be a stepping stone on your great journey toward abundant health and happiness. May you find the accountability you need to achieve all of your goals. May you awaken to find you have transformed into the success story version of yourself. May you give the gift of health and happiness to everyone you meet. Thank you for being a part of my journey and may our paths meet again.

ABOUT THE AUTHOR

Summer Peterson is known as Wine Country's leading weight loss expert who specializes in how to speed up your metabolism and turn on your skinny genes. Host of the television show, Wine Country Weight Loss with Summer Peterson and founder of BodySoulShine, she has developed online weight loss programs that result in consistent, lasting weight loss. Summer's own weight loss journey was the catalyst for creating the SEXY Diet. After years of yo-yo dieting, Summer discovered how to lose weight without deprivation and fixed her broken metabolism. She now passionately teaches the art of weight loss and metabolism health. Summer has a master's degree in psychology. She lives in the heart of the Northern California Wine Country with her husband and their two sons, Jude and Skyler.